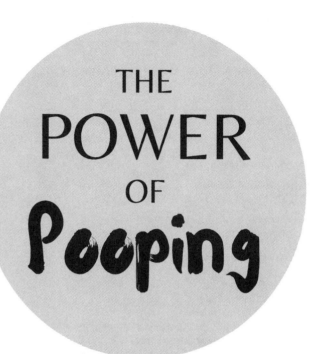

THE
POWER
OF
Pooping

**A Cheeky Diet and Lifestyle Guide to
End Constipation and Transform Your Health**

Nurse Wong
with John Rietcheck

Published by:
ULYSSES PRESS
PO Box 3440
Berkeley, CA 94703
www.ulyssespress.com

ISBN: 978-1-64604-265-4
Library of Congress Control Number: 2021937732

Printed in the United States by Versa Press
10 9 8 7 6 5 4 3 2 1

Acquisitions editor: Casie Vogel
Managing editor: Claire Chun
Editor: Renee Rutledge
Proofreader: Barbara Schultz
Front cover design: Katrina Yan
Interior design and layout: what!design @ whatweb.com
Production assistant: Yesenia Garcia-Lopez
Artwork: Julien Goavec

NOTE TO READERS: This book has been written and published for informational and educational purposes only. It is not intended to serve as medical advice or to be any form of medical treatment. You should always consult with your physician before altering or changing any aspect of your medical treatment. Do not stop or change any prescription medications without the guidance and advice of your physician. Any use of the information in this book is made on the reader's good judgment and is the reader's sole responsibility. This book is not intended to diagnose or treat any medical condition and is not a substitute for a physician. This book is independently authored and published, and no sponsorship or endorsement of this book by, and no affiliation with, any trademarked brands or other products mentioned within is claimed or suggested. All trademarks that appear in this book belong to their respective owners and are used here for informational purposes only. The author and publisher encourage readers to patronize the quality brands mentioned in this book.

To the silent sufferers who need guidance, treatment, and good old TLC to face and hopefully conquer the nasty poop-related issues that plague them every day.

—Susan Wong, aka Nurse Wong

CONTENTS

FOREWORD 7

INTRODUCTION 9

PART 1 15

CHAPTER 1 YOUR PLUMBING, FROM GUT TO BUTT 16

What Went Wrong? 19

The Power of Pooping. 21

What Is the Digestive System? 22

Gut-Brain Connections 24

Your Plumbing System 26

Your Gut Is the Home of Your Microbiome 31

The Healthy Human Plumbing System. 33

CHAPTER 2 HOW WELL DOES YOUR PLUMBING WORK?. 36

What's Up with Potty Training?. 40

Let's Open Up about Pooping Problems 41

How Is Your Pooping Process Working? 44

Poop Quiz 44

Nurse Wong's 3P Questionnaire (Pre-Poop, Poop, Post-Poop) 47

CHAPTER 3 CONSTIPATION AIN'T NO FUN! 60

A Little about Me and My Past Poop Problems. 63

Let's Talk Constipation 65

What Causes Constipation? 66

What Is the Prevalence of Chronic Constipation? 69

How Is Constipation Diagnosed?. 73

How Is Constipation Treated? **79**

Laxatives to Loosen Your Poop **82**

Supplements for Constipation Relief **84**

Biofeedback and Electrical Stimulation Therapy
(No, Not Shock Therapy!) **88**

Kegel Exercises **90**

Don't Give Up the Ship **90**

CHAPTER 4 KNOW THY FOOD **92**

Food in the 21st Century—How Did We Get Here? **94**

What Are Empty-Calorie Foods? **101**

Stay Hydrated! **104**

Fiber, Fiber, and More Fiber! **106**

Daily Fiber Recommendations **111**

What Other Healthy Foods Should I Eat? **113**

What about Sugar? **114**

Are Carbohydrates Bad for You? **115**

What Is a Recommended Healthy Diet? **117**

CHAPTER 5 TOOLS FOR THE PERFECT POOPING PROTOCOL . . . **120**

How to Properly Poop **125**

Review Your Supplements for Adverse Gut Effects **133**

Review Your Medications for Unwanted Side Effects **134**

CHAPTER 6 LIFESTYLE CHOICES FOR THE JOY OF POOPING . . . **136**

Good Diet—No Exercise **141**

Four Key Lifestyle Choices for Better Pooping **143**

Create Your Own Poop Schedule **149**

Motivation Is Your Key to Success **153**

CHAPTER 7 FEEL THE POWER OF POOPING! **155**

Closing Thoughts **163**

PART 2 165

CHAPTER 8 PREPARATIONS FOR EATING HEALTHY 166
Practical Tips for Eating on a Budget 167

CHAPTER 9 RECIPES FOR CONSTIPATION RELIEF. 179

Breakfast
Fruit Smoothies 182
Nurse Wong's Morning Staple: Oatmeal 185
Overnight Chia Seed Pudding. 187
Overnight Oats. 190
Muesli and Overnight Muesli 192

Lunch
Healthy Burrito with Brown Rice, Beans, and Chicken 196
Curried Cubed Chicken Salad. 200
Healthy PB&J Sandwich with Multigrain Bread 203
Chicken Noodle Vegetable Soup. 205
Tomato Mozzarella Basil Salad. 208

Dinner
Oven-Roasted Fish with Polenta and Vegetables 210
Roasted Lemon Herbed Chicken with Brown Rice and Veggies . . 213
Herb-Roasted Rack of Lamb with Baked Potatoes and Salad. . . . 217
Savory Meatless Cornmeal-Crust Pizza with Baked Figs. 222
Shrimp with Grains and Veggies 225
Week-at-a-Glance Meal Schedule and Table. 228

RESOURCES 233

ABOUT THE AUTHORS 237

FOREWORD

I have known Susan Wong for ten years and in that time, I have come to appreciate the depth of knowledge and dedication she brings to her chosen area of expertise: "the art and science of pooping." In the care of her patients, Susan is masterful in her analysis of complex clinical issues related to bowel function, and competent and kind in management of these problems.

In this book, she has compiled forty years of accumulated knowledge and wisdom into a volume that is practical and humorous. It incorporates concrete examples and facts. The general public will enjoy it and anyone with pooping problems will find it pragmatic and comprehensive.

For as long as I have known her, Susan's goal has been "to help people poop better." This book is a reflection of that and is a must read for anyone with interest in this topic.

Ankit Sarin, MD
Associate Professor
Colon and Rectal Surgery
University of California–San Francisco

INTRODUCTION

I've come a long way from my early childhood days, when my mother, newly immigrated from Hong Kong, applied her folk medicine remedies on me whenever I was "out of balance." In Cantonese, she would tell me that I was having *jit hei* (yeet hay), or "hot heat," which translates to "inflammation of the body." Whenever I was running a temperature and had a sore throat, she would cook me winter melon soup since my body "needed to be corrected from its inner heat" (the fever).

I didn't mind most of her ideas and folk treatments, but when it came time for my menstrual cycle, she told me that I couldn't wash my hair because that would create dark circles under my eyes. Well, I just couldn't swallow that one.

When I was fifteen years old, my maternal grandmother came to live with us. I got a greater insight into more of the old-school Chinese remedies and realized where my mother's beliefs and superstitions came from. I remember seeing a bottle of cognac and a cup of chrysanthemum tea on the nightstand by my grandmother's bed. At the time, I figured the cognac was to help her relax and get to sleep, but I had no idea what the tea was for. Later on, I discovered that chrysanthemum tea has medicinal properties for calming the gut, similar to chamomile.

When my grandmother felt like she was coming down with an illness, she would call her son-in-law, a surgeon trained in Western medicine, for advice. After getting, then promptly ignoring his recommendations, she immediately called her Chinese acupuncturist for his take, since she was more trusting of his advice. She even had a metal container of her own acupuncture needles that she took to her appointments with him. Being from the "old" country, she much preferred traditional Chinese medicine.

Although I was influenced by both my mother's and grand-mother's use of Eastern remedies during my formative years, the connection I had with my aunts, who were nurses and educators, spurred me toward a career in nursing. To this day, there's a place for both Eastern and Western medicine in my life.

In my clinical training to become a nurse, I realized how much I enjoyed working with patients and helping them in a variety of ways. There has never been a dull moment on the journey through my forty-three-year nursing career, which has taken me from pediatrics to adult medicine, dialysis, the operating room, and finally, the colorectal surgery department's subdi-vision of the Center of Pelvic Physiology. This is where I spent the last twenty-two years of my career, working with patients young and old from all walks of life, who suffered from some form of pelvic floor dysfunction. Their conditions ranged from a host of issues related to surgical recovery to a plethora of nonsurgical problems, all related to defecation.

At the Center of Pelvic Physiology, I worked closely with a team of specialists that included gastroenterologists, colorectal surgeons, nurse practitioners, physical therapists, and other health-care providers. Our collaboration was invaluable to me in the treatment of my patients, many of whom had very complex conditions.

I suppose it was my voracious appetite for learning, coupled with a strong desire to do everything possible to help my patients (sometimes outside of work hours), that led my coworkers to dub me "The Rear Admiral!"

When my son, Julien, proposed the idea of creating a YouTube channel with me as the "star," I thought he was kidding. I should have remembered; when he has an idea, he explores every angle, sets a goal, lays out the steps to achieve it, and digs in until it comes into fruition!

With the advent of *Butt Talks TV* and its rising popularity, a representative of Ulysses Press approached me to write this book. Honestly, once I accepted their offer and was faced with the reality of writing a book on poop health, I felt over-whelmed and a little inadequate. With the support of my family and friends, along with my wealth of experience, those feel-ings soon gave way to the realization that I had an incredible opportunity to reach many people who suffer in silence every day from embarrassing poop-related issues.

I want you all to meet Butty, the main character and mascot of *Butt Talks TV***, the flagship YouTube channel where I share practical information on everything poop-related. Butty happily and helpfully appears throughout the book in several sidenotes.**

On your journey through this book, you will discover that my approach to the pooping process is holistic and, oftentimes, humorous. I will touch upon the relationship between science, psychology, mindfulness, the economics of diet, and cultural and social dietary practices, as well as giving you practical tips for better poop health.

Despite an abundance of facts, figures, and remedies readily available on the information highway, many people just like you and me are confused about to how to deal with their pooping problems. Constipation, fecal incontinence, or one of a multitude of other maladies may plague you, family members, friends, or coworkers. Most likely you suffer in silence, reticent to share your condition, even with close confidants.

Eating and pooping involve multifactorial processes that the general public, as well as those who suffer poop-related issues, often misunderstand.

To paraphrase William Ernest Henley's famous poem "Invictus," the bottom line is that you are the master of your fate, the captain of your soul. You can fill your brain with tons of information, but until you parse out what meaningfully relates to your individual circumstances and take action to help yourself, you are simply biding your time.

The information in these pages may not solve all your poop-related problems because we are all individuals with different needs and unique situations. However, it will provide guidance and practical approaches to help you manage and hopefully resolve your poopy problems though education, lifestyle changes, and simple, everyday recipes.

I am grateful for the opportunity to help you, the reader, and so many of the people I serve, to conquer your demons and learn to manage your poop health. As I often say to my patients and coworkers alike, "everyone has to poop, so let's put them in poop heaven."

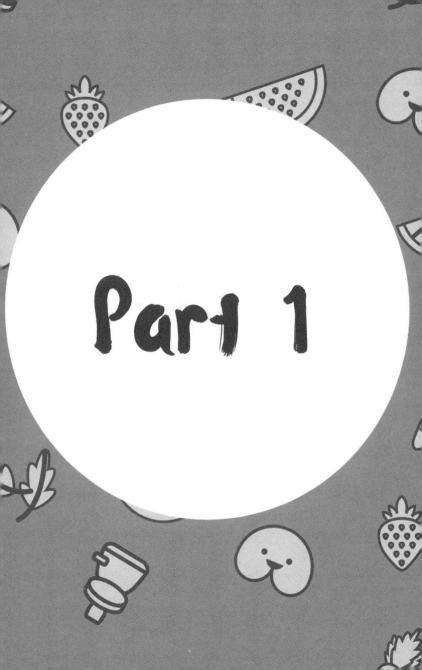

CHAPTER 1

YOUR PLUMBING, FROM GUT TO BUTT

"Should I refuse a good dinner simply because I do not understand the process of digestion?"

—Oliver Heaviside[1]

ELLA'S STORY: DOING ALL THE WRONG THINGS

Ella, a single, thirty-something, stressed-out, multitasking manager of a software start-up, wakes up with a jolt, looks at her phone, and realizes she has overslept. It is Wednesday, and today of all days, she can't be late for work since she's in charge of a team meeting. She throws on her clothes, drags a comb through her tangled hair, and heads for the

---

1. Oliver Heaviside, *Electromagnetic Theory*, vol. 2 (London: Electrician Printing and Publishing Co, 1899), 9.

kitchen. Once in the kitchen, she grabs the large cinnamon roll her coworker gave her yesterday at work, nukes it, then ferociously attacks it. She washes down the sweet, doughy mixture in her mouth with a cup of day-old coffee she didn't even bother to heat, grabs her coat and purse, rushes out the door and off to work.

Ella is lucky that the traffic isn't snarled, so she arrives with six minutes to spare. Once at work, she immediately heads to the employee lounge, pours herself a 32-ounce cup of hot black coffee and heads to the conference room for the meeting.

The meeting goes swimmingly.

But now, with a ton of tasks to finish before the day ends, Ella knocks back the rest of her coffee. By 11:00 a.m. she feels the heartburn creeping up her throat, so she pops a couple of chewable antacids and gets back to work. Since there's so much on her plate today, Ella skips lunch to keep up with the day's to-do list. She finally takes a short break around 3:00 p.m. There are a couple of large slices of pepperoni pizza in a box sitting on the counter in the lounge, so she picks one up and quickly gobbles it down cold, chasing it with yet another large cup of black coffee.

Since she stayed focused and completed her tasks for the day, Ella is able to leave work at 5:00 p.m. for a change. It isn't until she gets home that she realizes her stomach is rumbling. This leads her to a further realization: although she peed several times, she hasn't pooped all day. Not one to let little things like the lack of a bowel movement or a mild tummy ache bother her, she heads to the gym and works out for almost an hour.

After her workout, Ella finally feels like she might be able to poop. She gets situated on the toilet and waits a couple of minutes. When nothing happens, she pushes hard to get the process going. When just a few small, round turds plop into the water, she sighs, then pushes harder to try to open the poop gates. More small turds come out. Eventually, Ella decides she has pooped enough, so she vigorously wipes her butt until there's a little blood mixed with the poop on the toilet paper, which is normal for her.

After a well-deserved hot shower, Ella orders dinner through Uber Eats. When it arrives, the aroma wafting from the exquisitely textured lasagna, antipasto, breadsticks, and marinara sauce tantalizes Ella's senses. She pours a glass of cabernet sauvignon and digs in. After the main course, she eats a slice of New York–style cheesecake. Ella has eaten so much that she feels more stuffed than she has in a very long time. She smiles to herself at what a great day she had! But before calling it a night, she impulsively decides to binge-watch a series that everyone is talking about at work. By the time she finishes, it is 1:00 a.m. As she performs her nightly routine

THE POWER OF **Pooping**

before bed, she feels the acid rising up her throat again, but this time the heartburn is more intense. Ella takes three ant-acids and goes to bed.

WHAT WENT WRONG?

Ella's story, though fictional, mimics that of thousands of real-life people I've seen over the course of my career as the "Rear Admiral." Ella thinks she had a great day, but let's explore where that isn't true. For starters, she is stressed out from oversleeping, which has her nerve endings frayed. The half-chewed, fiberless, high-fat, empty-calorie sweet roll goes down her throat as a lump of dough and sugar while the coffee acts as a bladder irritant, removing water from her body via her frequent pee breaks. The result is dehydration.

After Ella's day of poor eating and drinking, she suffers the consequences of her actions. Hard-charging, type-A Ella is *constipated*! Too much coffee, cold pizza, and later, more fiberless, high-fat food with dehydrating alcohol created heartburn twice because of their acidic qualities and her lack of hydration. The antacids act only as temporary Band-Aids masking the symptoms of her heartburn. Her grumbling stomach is another sign that Ella's gut is out of whack. The dehydration withdraws water from her colon (large intestine), making the stools hard and dry.

She makes things worse by pushing and straining to poop (this is very bad, by the way) for a small yield of a few hard, dry popcorn turds, followed by obsessive wiping (which is also bad), until she draws blood from her abused anus. Ella, in turn, doesn't get enough sleep. Sleep would help her body recharge as well as protect her from disease.

BUTTY'S SIDENOTE

For those of us who consume fiber-rich foods and drink plenty of water, one cup of coffee in the morning can stimulate the smooth muscles of the large intestine to facilitate your first poop of the day. If your daily regimen consists of limited amounts of fiber and water plus several cups of strong coffee, you may very well end up with lots of pee breaks, few, if any, poops, and the caffeine jitters to boot.

Now, let's not get all bound up with constipation (pun intended) right now; in later chapters, I plan to delve deeper into constipation, along with other related issues like dehydration and fiberless foods. But for now, whether you realized it before or not, you can see that understanding the power of pooping could truly change Ella's (and your) life!

THE POWER OF POOPING

When most people put food or drink in their mouths, they are clueless about the magic or, in Ella's case, the mayhem, that can happen as it slides down the esophagus to the stomach, traverses 30 feet of small and large intestines to the poop chute, the rectum, and out of the anus after twenty-four to forty hours. As the late motivational speaker Jim Rohn once said, "Treat your body like a temple, not a woodshed. The mind and body work together. Your body needs to be a good support system for the mind and spirit."[2]

I firmly believe that if people understood the basic anatomy and function of the components in their digestive system, they would not treat their bodies like a woodshed but with more love, kindness, and respect. When I'm working in the clinic, I often explain to my patients that the digestive system is truly an intricately designed network of plumbing that only works well when it isn't clogged with an accumulation of cluttered waste. My job is to act as the master plumber to help them become mindful enough of the digestive process to make positive

2.   Jim Rohn, "The Treasury of Quotes," Open Library, Health Communications, September 1, 1996, https://openlibrary.org/books/OL8607826M/The_Treasury_of_Quotes, 49.

changes to their diets and lifestyles. Only then can they fully realize the true power of pooping!

WHAT IS THE DIGESTIVE SYSTEM?

Now, let's take the plunge to plumb the depths of your plumbing. As the supersleuth Sherlock Holmes might say, "It's 'alimentary,' my dear Watson." The alimentary or gastrointestinal tract (GI, for short) includes the mouth, throat, esophagus, stomach, small intestine, large intestine, rectum, and anus. The pancreas, gall bladder, and liver are also important components of the digestive system. That may sound like a lot to swallow, but you don't have to be a scientist or a plumber to be familiar with the parts of your digestive system. As Sir Francis Bacon said back in the 16th century, "Knowledge is power." In this case, knowledge is pooping power!

Now that you know a little about the anatomy of your plumbing system, let's take a closer look at how your pipes connect and work together. You may remember an old song about your bones: "The thigh bone's connected to the knee bone," etc. Just like your skeleton, everything in your digestive system is also connected (although part of it is pretty kinky), and each part has a specific function: to get the food you eat to pass from one section to another down the labyrinth of those 30 feet of intestines to the poop chute. The overall purpose of your digestive system is to transform the food you put in your body into rich nutrients that provide you with energy, cellular repair, and growth.

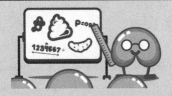

WITH PROFESSOR BUTTY'S HELP, LET'S START AT THE BEGINNING.

Even before you put food in your mouth, your sight and sense of smell have triggered your salivary glands to start the juices flowing in anticipation of enjoying the grub you will soon eat. Saliva helps with digestion, wets your mouth, reduces infection in your mouth and throat, and provides protection to your teeth and gums. Emotionally, you may feel elated, grateful, or even possessive of what you are about to consume. If you are with family or friends, the good food and company might spark a little laughter as you all prepare to partake in the shared culinary delights.

GUT-BRAIN CONNECTIONS

During and after your meal, your central nervous system is sending and receiving messages of rich dialogue between the one hundred million (give or take a few thousand) nerve cells of your enteric nervous system (ENS), which is embedded in the walls of your gut and controls spontaneous movement of waste, blood flow, and nutrient absorption. Sympathetic nerves, part of the "autonomic," or involuntary nervous system, act to accelerate your heart rate, slow down the muscle movement of your large intestine, constrict blood vessels, and increase wavelike contractions that move food along the digestive tract (a process called "peristalsis"). The sympathetic nerves in the esophagus branch out from the gut to the spinal cord, then on to the brain stem, which regulates your basic bodily functions.

The parasympathetic nerve network, sometimes called the "rest-and-digest nerves," is also part of the autonomic system. It serves to counterbalance the sympathetic nerves by conserving energy while slowing your heart rate, increasing the activity of the intestines and glands, and allowing your sphincter muscles to efficiently facilitate peaceful, easy pooping.

These two nerve networks transmit signals to and from the brain stem via the vagus nerve from the colon. In one of his feeble attempts at humor, my anatomy and physiology professor in college told us that if we couldn't find the vagus nerve on a chart of the human anatomy, we were required to call it the "lost vagus" nerve. All dad jokes aside, the vagus nerve is the most prominent pathway connecting the brain to the gut. In fact, it runs from the brain through the lungs, heart, spleen, liver, and kidneys all the way to the intestines and your microbiome, which you will soon learn about.

Both the gut and the brain utilize shared neurotransmitters, acetylcholine and neuropeptides (chemicals stimulating nerve signal transmissions), to send information back and forth. This bidirectional messaging system lets you know when you are full or, conversely, when anxiety curbs your appetite, as Ella experienced.

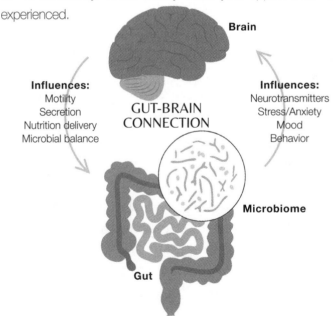

Brain

Influences:
Motility
Secretion
Nutrition delivery
Microbial balance

GUT-BRAIN CONNECTION

Influences:
Neurotransmitters
Stress/Anxiety
Mood
Behavior

Microbiome

Gut

The diagram above will give you a better idea of this all-important bidirectional system.

YOUR PLUMBING SYSTEM

Now, back to the important way stations along your plumbing system. Once you put that first bite of food in your mouth, the average ten thousand taste buds on your tongue wake up and say, "Howdy-do!" which allows you to experience the unique flavors of food and drink: sweet, salty, sour, and bitter, as well as combinations of each.

Chewing, combined with the enzymatic action of amylase and lingua lipase in your saliva, starts to break down the food. The amylase helps break down the starches (carbohydrates) into sugars, while the lipase breaks down the fats so your body can more easily absorb the food. The importance of chewing is often overlooked by eaters like Ella, who stuffs chunks of cinnamon roll in her mouth without thoroughly breaking it down, expecting the coffee to help it along. She's lucky the partially chewed roll with the coffee chaser went down her throat to the esophagus, the muscular tube that delivers food to her stomach, rather than the "wrong pipe," the windpipe. Unfortunately, we've all suffered the consequences of the repugnant regurgitative reactions that follow! Let's take a look at the digestive system using the diagram here:

THE POWER OF **Pooping**

DIGESTIVE SYSTEM

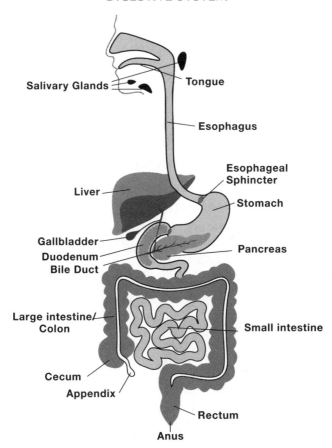

As you can easily see, the digestive system has many parts. I don't want to get too academic here so I'll do my best to keep it as clear as possible.

Station 1: The esophagus. Once you swallow your well-chewed food, it slides down the esophagus, where peristalsis moves it along toward the stomach. There's a valve at the lower part of the esophagus called the esophageal sphincter (you see, it really is a plumbing system) that pushes the food into the stomach and keeps it from going backward in the wrong direction. (It can and does go backward when we're sick and we upchuck, vomit, hurl…well, you get what I mean.) Once the food is in your stomach, the strong muscular lining holds it and does a bump and grind dance to mix it up. Your stomach secretes acid and powerful enzymes that continue to break the food down into a liquid-like paste until it passes into your small intestine.

Station 2: The small intestine. Your small intestine is a very long, coiled tube in the abdomen. Amazingly, if it were spread out in a straight line, it would be about 20 feet long! Your small intestine continues the process of breaking down food using more enzymes released from the pancreas, along with bile from the liver and gallbladder. Bile helps with the digestion and absorption of fats and removes waste products from the blood. Again, peristalsis occurs in the small intestine, moving the food along as it mixes with digestive secretions. Important components of your small intestine continue to break down the food and eventually facilitate absorption of the nutrients into your bloodstream.

Station 3: The gallbladder. This pear-shaped organ serves as a storage receptacle for the bile that comes from the liver through the hepatic duct. The gallbladder sends bile to the beginning of the small intestine called the duodenum via the common bile duct.

Station 4: The large intestine. Your large intestine, or colon, is a muscular tube from 5 to 6 feet long, with a larger diameter than the small intestine. It has many interconnected parts, which I'll break down separately below.

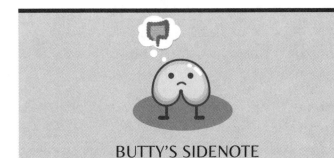

BUTTY'S SIDENOTE

We've got about 6 feet of intestine to go before we get to what I call the "poop chute," or rectum. If this material is a bit dry for you, please drink plenty of water to stay hydrated because you'll need it to cross the finish line!

Station 5: The cecum (pronounced see-come). The first part of your colon is the cecum, a pouch-like structure at the juncture of the small and large intestines. The cecum acts as a reservoir for a pulpy, acidic fluid (called chyme and pronounced *kime*), consisting of gastric juices and partially digested food that mix with the mucous lining in the walls of the cecum. The cecum also absorbs fluids and salts that remain after digestion in the small intestine.

Stations 6 to 8: The ascending, transverse, and descending sections of the colon. After the cecum, your colon rises (ascending) from the right and crosses to the left side of your body (transverse section). From there it descends (descending section) and delivers waste down to the S-shaped (sigmoid) area that connects to the poop chute (rectum). Again, in all these sections, the process of peristalsis continues after the waste is delivered from the small intestine to the cecum.

Station 9: The rectum. Your colon works to reabsorb fluids and process the waste to form stool that is stored in the S-shaped area until you feel (that is, if your plumbing system isn't clogged) what I call "the Urge." The Urge, or "mass movement," occurs when there's enough poop in the rectum to stretch and expand it. Once it is sufficiently stretched, the pelvic floor muscles of the anus, along with the two amazing anal sphincters, begin to do their magic. An angle between the rectum and the anus is created by the pelvic floor muscles, keeping poop from being expelled at the wrong time, like when we are sleeping. Thank goodness for that!

When the poop reaches the internal anal sphincter, the defecation reflex kicks in, signaling the internal muscle of the anal sphincter to relax and the external anal sphincter (a skeletal muscle you have some control over) to contract. The finely tuned motor control of your pelvic floor muscles, along with the internal and external anal sphincter muscles usually (but not always) prevent us from the mess and embarrassment of pooping in our pants!

The end result of this exquisite network of living organic tissue in your gut-to-butt plumbing system is that when you reach the finish line, if you are in good poop health, you will experience the cathartic moment of release when the poop easily comes out of your wonderfully awesome anus. That's when you truly feel the power of pooping!

YOUR GUT IS THE HOME OF YOUR MICROBIOME

You may or may not realize that I left out a mere forty trillion inhabitants of your gut, mostly residing in the cecum, the pouch at the beginning of your colon. Collectively, they are called your "gut microbiome." No, they aren't alien monsters that suddenly emerge from your belly and do a little dance. They are microscopic bacterial, viral, and fungal cells, or microbes that I call the "good gut guys," as opposed to the "bad gut guys," the bacteria that can make you sick. In reality, there are more microbial cells in your body than the approximately 30 trillion human cells.

And, according to the National Institutes of Health, there are as many as one thousand species of the good gut guys living in your body, all with different functions.

If there were a way to collect all these good gut guys and put them on a scale, they might weigh anywhere from 2 to 5 pounds total! Working as a team, these good microbes act as an additional organ in your body and play a major role in your overall health.

WHO ARE THE GOOD GUT GUYS, AND WHAT DO THEY DO?

As humans have evolved over millions of years, the body has adapted to living with microbes. And microbes have come to play such a critical part in the health of our bodies that without them, we might not survive.

Your gut microbiome began to have an effect on your body the day you traversed your mother's birth canal. Based on a 2017 *Nature Medicine* article, there is also evidence that babies come in contact with some microbes while still in the womb.[3]

---

3. Derrick M. Chu et al., "Maturation of the Infant Microbiome Community Structure and Function across Multiple Body Sites and in Relation to Mode of Delivery," *Nature Medicine* 23, no. 3 (2017): 314–26, https://doi.org/10.1038/nm.4272.

After you were born and your body began to grow, your gut microbiome branched out, adding many varied species of microbes. The greater the diversity of these good gut guys, the healthier you tend to be.

Good gut bacteria help you digest fiber that produces short-chain fatty acids, contributing to the prevention of weight gain, heart disease, cancer, and diabetes. Your good gut guys also help regulate your immune system and respond to infections. Last but not least, a 2012 article in *Nature Reviews Neuroscience* found strong indications that your microbiome, via your central nervous system, may contribute to mood changes, anxiety, pain, and cognition as well as your overall brain health in response to stress.[4]

THE HEALTHY HUMAN PLUMBING SYSTEM

In the first installment of Ella's story (you guessed it, her story is far from over), you saw how poor choices of food and drink, coupled with a stressful lifestyle, created a cesspool in her clogged plumbing system. We know that an unhealthy gut can lead to a variety of diseases that include obesity, diabetes, depression, rheumatoid arthritis, and chronic fatigue.

4.   John F. Cryan and Timothy G. Dinan, "Mind-Altering Microorganisms: The Impact of the Gut Microbiota on Brain and Behaviour," *Nature Reviews Neuroscience*, September 12, 2012, https://doi.org/10.1038/nrn3346.

That begs the question: What does a healthy human plumbing system look like?

In order to promote a healthy gut, it's important to have at least a basic understanding of how your plumbing system works.

In a nutshell, your digestive system serves to break down liquids and foods into the chemical components of carbohydrates, fats, and proteins for your body to absorb using the extracted nutrients for energy, cell growth, and repair.

A healthy plumbing system produces beneficial digestive enzymes along with a rich, varied microbiome of the good gut guys to do the following effectively and efficiently:

- absorb vital nutrients
- prevent the growth of the bad gut guys that lead to disease
- eliminate toxins and other foreign substances from the body

If you have a healthy digestive system, you process the food you eat in around twenty-four to forty hours (depending on your plumbing system) and pass the waste material easily and efficiently in one to two bowel movements of full-bodied, smooth stools per day. The consistency, shape, and color of your stools are a reflection of your health—that includes your diet, how hydrated you are, the medications you use, and possible medical conditions you may have. I will illustrate the types of healthy vs. unhealthy stools via Nurse Wong's Poop Pictogram on page 72.

It's fascinating to me that over two thousand years ago, Hippocrates, the Greek physician, was onto something when he said, "all disease begins in the gut." With the multitude of diet plans (some helpful, some just bad fads) overpopulating the internet, libraries, and bookstores, it's no wonder people are confused as to what they need to do to foster a clean, well-functioning plumbing system. As your master plumber, I will provide simple tips to help you sort out what you can do to create a better life and healthier plumbing system through diet, lifestyle, and medical intervention, when necessary.

CHAPTER 2

HOW WELL DOES YOUR PLUMBING WORK?

"I have finally cum to the konklusion that a good reliable set ov bowels iz worth more to a man than enny quantity of brains."
—Josh Billings, pen name of Henry Wheeler Shaw, 19th-century humorist

ELLA'S STORY: FROM BAD TO WORSE

Ella wakes up with a start when her Big Ben cell phone alarm goes off at 6:30 a.m. She hits the snooze button every ten minutes until 7:30 a.m., leaving only thirty minutes for her to get up and get ready for work. Ella feels exhausted, and her stomach hurts. Her 120-pound body feels as if it weighs 300 pounds as she slowly climbs out of bed and finds her way to the coffee pot to make that all-important shot of strong wake-up juice.

With a large cup full of warm black coffee in hand, she makes her way to the bathroom, sits on the porcelain throne, cell phone in hand, and downs half the java while checking her emails and trying to poop. She strains and pushes hard in hopes of having a big poop to ease the pressure in her gut. Not a single tiny turd comes out. Instead, she pees like a horse emptying her bladder, which seems to provide a bit of relief to her abdomen. After five minutes she gives up on having a morning poop-fest and decides to take a quick shower in hopes of becoming more alert. After showering and dressing, she takes the leftover lasagna from the fridge, cuts a large piece, and anxiously consumes half of it cold. Ella then packs the remaining chunk of lasagna in a sealed container for her lunch. She's in such a rush that she doesn't notice that the socks she put on don't even come close to matching! Type-A Ella actually relishes the challenge of getting ready for work in record time. The anxiety triggers adrenaline to rapidly course through her body, giving her a burst of energy.

Ella makes it to work twelve minutes late. With a looming deadline, the office soon becomes a pressure cooker of angst. A couple of other managers get into a shouting match. It isn't long before most of the support staff are walking on eggshells, hunching over their open-design workstations whenever a manager is in close proximity. Ella, trying not to get caught up in this menagerie of mental anguish, tries to encourage her team the best she knows how, then hunkers down to the work at hand while unconsciously internalizing the stress into every fiber of her being.

With so much to accomplish before the deadline, Ella doesn't eat anything other than a small amount of micro-waved popcorn her assistant gave her. She manages to generate more get-up-and-go energy by drinking two cups of espresso midmorning and guzzling a can of energy drink that afternoon. By late evening, Ella begins to feel extreme fatigue washing over her. Finally leaving work after twelve hours of nonstop mental exertion, Ella realizes her entire body, from head to shoulders to legs to toes, is knotted up and sore. She has a stiff neck and a headache, as well as an upset stomach. She doesn't feel particularly hungry but knows she should eat something. It doesn't even dawn on her that she hasn't pooped all day.

With the deadline fast approaching, Ella works grueling over-time for nine straight days. Her days become eerily similar. She gets four to five hours of sleep each night, drinks lots of coffee and energy drinks during the day, and starts eating TV dinners and fast food most nights after work to save time.

Some nights she is so tired and stressed that she drinks a bottle of Coke and eats a handful of potato chips—or nothing at all. She becomes acutely aware that her stomach constantly hurts and her abdomen is pooched out. The most significant nonevent coinciding with her upset stomach and distended abdomen is that she has not pooped once during the entire nine-day period. This is when Ella really begins to worry about her health.

She no longer shrugs it off when she can't poop, despite pushing and straining every day she sits on the pot. She has no doubt that she is seriously constipated. She reads a few online articles about constipation and how it can lead to bowel blockages for which medical intervention, hospitalization, and, sometimes, surgeries are necessary. Ella starts to get frightened, so frightened that she calls her mom in tears and everything spills out: her constipation and associated health-related fears, the stress of her toxic work environment, and a host of other simmering stressors rising to the surface, threatening to boil over and burn her badly.

We'll get back to Ella's story in the next chapter. As I mentioned before, her story is the same or similar to that of many of my patients. I often wonder, How and when did all their problems begin? Some patients tell me it started when they were small children.

WHAT'S UP WITH POTTY TRAINING?

What in the world does potty training have to do with the current state of your plumbing system? We typically begin to develop bowel and bladder control when we are between twenty-four and forty-eight months old, give or take a few months. Toilet training, whether done in a positive or negative way, is one of the most important times of anyone's young life. Being diaper-free is a true milestone in the development of greater independence and self-esteem for any toddler. If your parents' attitudes were to pressure and/or shame you during potty training, then your early toileting experiences may have led to unhealthy habits and behaviors that have continued throughout your life.

Some of my patients tell me that they were always rushed to poop and pee during potty training because several other members of the household needed to use the toilet too. So, they either learned to hold it back and ignore the feeling until it was gone, or to wait so long that when they finally had a chance to go, they had difficulty fully emptying the poop or pee from their little bodies.

Others felt they were pressured to produce throughout the training process by their parents or caretakers, who were not patient and caring enough to wait for them to do their business within a reasonable amount of time. Some of them were not given the privacy, comfort, and positive feedback to feel successful about their toileting experiences. I often see the connection between my patients' childhood potty issues and their current condition. Some of them still feel as if they don't have enough time or privacy to "do their thing."

LET'S OPEN UP ABOUT POOPING PROBLEMS

I wrote this book because I truly want to help people live their best lives. Every day I listen to my patients and read the email comments from *Butt Talks TV* viewers telling me about all the doubts and emotional distress they have around their pooping problems.

We as a society are not very open or comfortable discussing the messy topic of our poop problems with immediate family or clinically driven doctors who, on average, spend a mere five to seven minutes face to face with us. Some of my patients harbor such pervasive fears and attached emotions toward a poop problem that they ultimately fall down the rabbit hole of the internet. They really don't want to go there, but sometimes they feel as if they have nowhere else to turn for help or advice. And, despite the abundance of resources online on poop health, sometimes it is too general, or not applicable to their needs, or they simply don't know where to begin.

My patients have taught me that their greatest need is to see a provider who can make them feel comfortable sharing their poop secrets *and*, most importantly, listen to them with compassion. I have taken that to heart, so gaining their trust by listening and connecting compassionately with them as human beings is my number one priority. One way I accomplish this is by directly involving them in the process of the various tests I perform, which includes prompting them to squeeze and release their pelvic floor muscles along with several other tasks, and telling me what sensations they are feeling. I also make sure to explain, in layman's terms, the results of each test, along with the positive or negative functionality of their pelvic floor muscles. I have found that my patients become much more invested in their own poop health when they are included in the process. This, in turn, makes them more likely to listen to me when I share important self-help tools and techniques to help them resolve their issues.

As you've undoubtedly figured out by now, we all have pooping problems at various stages in our lives. Those issues are often easily resolved via over-the-counter medicines or small changes in diet. Unfortunately, for many of us, pooping problems have been unwelcome companions in our world for many months, years, or decades. The longer these problems persist, the more likely you are to pick up coping mechanisms in the form of bad habits. My many years as a "poopatologist" (my self-created name for what I do) have shown me that when a long-term poop problem impacts your quality of life, expert medical treatment from a compassionate provider can go a long way to help you resolve and/or manage chronic conditions. Depending on the gravity of your specific issue, it will likely take a fair amount of time and a lot of conscious effort to make the changes that will get you and your pooping back to some semblance of normalcy.

There are as many ideas on how to approach healthy pooping as there are shades of color in the produce section of the supermarket. If you have serious long-term poop issues, the guidance of an excellent health practitioner can help you find the options that most closely agree with your lifestyle, or that at least give you the flexibility to change your unhealthy habits for the best possible outcome. The following information and fun self-assessments of your plumbing system can be quite helpful in getting you started on opening up about your pooping problems.

HOW IS YOUR POOPING PROCESS WORKING?

Let's take a look at some easy ways to explore the current status of your gut and your poop health in particular. I've already given you some basic information related to your plumbing system and its functions, which should help you as we move ahead.

I love to give poop quizzes! They are a great way to test your knowledge of how you fit into the poop loop. (Relax, this is the School of Poopatology, so you won't be graded.)

Poop Quiz

---

1. How many times should I poop each day?

    a. zero to one

    b. once

    c. twice

    d. three times

2. My poop should always be brown because that means I'm healthy.

☐ True   ☐ False

3. How long does it take food to traverse my plumbing system before I poop it out?

    a. 4 to 6 hours

    b. 8 to 10 hours

    c. 12 to 16 hours

    d. 20+ hours

4. My poop should always have an S-like shape.

    ☐ True   ☐ False

5. I should not have to push hard to get the poop out.

    ☐ True   ☐ False

6. How much time should I sit on the pot to poop?

    a. 2 minutes

    b. 5 to 10 minutes

    c. 15 minutes

    d. 20 minutes

7. Texting or making calls from my cell phone on the pot will not relax me.

    ☐ True   ☐ False

8. What's in my poop to make it float like a boat?

    a. Fat

    b. Fiber

    c. Gas

    d. Soda

9. If I'm an average person, I should pass gas (fart) about how many times a day?

    a. 2 to 4

    b. 8 to 9

    c. 12 to 14

    d. 20 to 40

10. Whether I'm healthy or not, my poop should typically stink.

    ☐ True   ☐ False

Answers: (1. A, 2. F, 3. D, 4. F, 5. T, 6. B, 7. T, 8. C, 9. C, 10. T)

I hope that you were able to get 70 to 80 percent of the Poop Quiz correct. If not, don't worry, because in the School of Poopatology, we give you the correct answers to help you learn and move a little further into the healthy poop loop.

One way I gather information about my patients' poop health relative to regularity vs. constipation is to have them complete Nurse Wong's 3P Questionnaire. Why don't you fill out the one below to get an idea of where you stand or, should I say, sit?

Nurse Wong's 3P Questionnaire (Pre-Poop, Poop, Post-Poop)

For this questionnaire, I will assess the quality of your poop from several varied aspects. This questionnaire has three sections: Pre-poop, Poop, and Post-poop. I will explain the significance of the questions after each section.

Please circle the number to the right of each answer so you can tally your score when finished.

PRE-POOP

1. Do you get a type of signal; a feeling or sound coming from your abdomen/stomach or from the end of your butt before you have to poop?

    a. Never (**1**)

    b. Sometimes (**2**)

    c. Always (**3**)

2. Do you end up peeing, pooping, or farting when you get these signals?

    a. Never (**1**)

    b. Sometimes (**2**)

    c. Always (**3**)

3. Do you find the poop sensation growing in intensity after you eat or drink, or during or after physical movement, even when sitting to standing?

    a. Never (**1**)

    b. Sometimes (**2**)

    c. Always (**3**)

4. Do you feel stronger poop sensations when you sit down or squat over the toilet?

    a. Never (**1**)

    b. Sometimes (**2**)

    c. Always (**3**)

5. During a typical one-week period, how many times do you actually poop?

    a. Less than once per week (**1**)

    b. Twice or less per week (**2**)

    c. Five or more times per week (**3**)

Add the numbers you circled for your Pre-Poop Score:

5 to 8   Uh-Oh!

9 to 12   So-So!

13 to 15   Hooray! You Go-Go! 😊 😊 💩

NURSE WONG'S NOTES ON THE PRE-POOP

Signal. The first question indicates how your body receives the signal to poop. Typically, you should have sensations of rectal pressure that let you know it's coming. If you score low on this question, it means that either your gut moves slowly, or there are some problems with the nerves that receive the signals (this is a more extreme case) as in someone who has suffered a spinal injury.

Response. The second question is a follow-up to the first. After receiving the signal, your body should react with corresponding results, like pooping or peeing. After you poop or pee, the sensation or the pressure should go away.

Motility. Similarly, for the third question, your body should be responsive to certain inputs like drinking or eating. Motility, or gut movement, is happening, and your body is preparing to have a poop soon! Usually, this is a great sign that your body is readily responsive. However, if your body is not as responsive, it's not the end of the world. When you get the urge, don't hold back the feeling very long. Make sure you get to the bathroom ASAP, or it will be more difficult to relax your muscles to poop later. Sometimes the poop feeling may disappear and you might skip a day. This could possibly put you in a constipated "danger zone," where you develop hard little stools that are difficult to pass.

Posture. Question four relates to the importance of posture. Think of your poop going down a slide; the poop angle must be just right so it can slide faster out of your butt! Correct posture should help your anal/rectal muscles relax and provide the optimal angle for the poop to come out more easily. We'll talk more about the posture and angles in Chapter 5.

Frequency. Question five is unique to each individual. Ideally, you will feel better if you poop every day. Just like having a morning coffee, daily poop is a welcoming feeling that makes you feel lighter, airier, relieved, and happy. You should feel good about your little daily routine. Some people have slower gut motility, so it could be once every two days, but that should be fine as long as the poop comes out soft and easy. If you poop less than twice a week or if your stools come out hard and painful over a several-week period, then the reasons why should be explored by you and your health professional.

POOP

1. How hard do you push to poop?

    a. Very hard—feels like the stool is stuck at the opening (**1**)

    b. Moderate—push occasionally (**2**)

    c. Not at all—no need to push, the stool just glides out smoothly (**3**)

2. Does it feel painful when the poop is coming out?

    a. Very painful (**1**)

    b. Moderately painful (**2**)

    c. No pain at all (**3**)

3. Do you feel comfortable sitting on the toilet to poop, or is it difficult to empty?

    a. Pooping is an unpleasant experience. I'm anxious and have to strain. (**1**)

    b. Pooping is somewhat difficult and unpleasant. (**2**)

    c. I feel relaxed and comfortable when I poop. (**3**)

4. How does your poop appear when you are not taking laxatives?

    a. Separate hard lumps, like nuts (**0**)

    b. Sausage-like but lumpy (**1**)

    c. Like a sausage but with cracks in the surface (**3**)

    d. Smooth, banana-shaped, and soft (**3**)

    e. Soft chunks with clear-cut edges (**2**)

    f. Mushy, with small fluffy pieces (**2**)

    g. Liquid, with no form (**1**)

5. Typically, how long do you spend on the toilet when pooping?

    a. 30 minutes or greater (**1**)

    b. 10 to 29 minutes (**2**)

    c. Less than10 minutes (**3**)

Your Poop Score:

5 to 8	Uh-Oh!
9 to 12	So-So!
13 to 15	Hooray! You Go-Go!

NURSE WONG'S NOTES ON THE POOP

Pushing. The first question is about pushing, which should not be necessary. Pooping should be natural and easy. If the pressure is there, your muscles have the right tension, and your poop has a soft, smooth texture, then it should slide easily out of your blueberry butthole.

Pushing, unfortunately, is a learned behavior. You may have been taught to push at an early age and, if this became a habit, you may now have problems relaxing on the toilet. (I will elaborate on this issue in Chapter 3).

Think about how your anus works—the more you push and strain it, the tighter it gets and the harder it is for anything to pass through. I cannot emphasize enough the importance of relaxing on the toilet. If you have to push, gently push only a few times, and let the muscle and gravity do the rest of the work.

Pain. Similarly for the second question, there should not be any pain during pooping. If you experience pain, it may be from extreme butt tension or muscle strain. If there's also blood in your poop, it might indicate a fissure or hemorrhoid.

Relaxation. Question three is all about comfort. To relax when pooping, some of my tips are:

1. Pretend you are blowing a feather to regulate your breathing, expand your diaphragm, and drop your pelvic muscles.

2. Use the warm spray from a bidet water jet, if available, to directly relax your anus.

3. Bring your knees up by putting your feet to a slightly elevated level to correct your butt angle.

Texture. Question four is all about paying attention to the texture of your turds. Poops should be soft and easy, like frozen yogurt or a nice ripe banana coming out of your butt. If your choices are not (c) or (d), you may need to fix your diet (monitor your fiber and fat intake), take away certain medications, and stay better hydrated. This will be a trial-and-error period, but do not give up. Instead, be consistent by observing your body and recording your habits for at least a couple of weeks.

Length. Question five is a follow-up to number four. If your poops slide out easily like frozen yogurt, you don't need much time on the pot. Usually, you should poop for ten minutes or less. Don't think that you need to sit on the toilet longer if nothing is coming out after ten minutes. It's just not going to happen—you aren't waiting for a bus. The best way to help get the poop out is to stand up, move around, and get hydrated (especially by drinking a warm beverage)—these actions can stimulate your gut to move (gastrocolic reflex).

POST-POOP

1. How many sheets of toilet paper do you use after your poop?

    a. The whole roll! (**1**)

    b. Many squares and repetitive wipes (**2**)

    c. Few squares and one or two wipes (**3**)

2. Do you see blood on your poop or on the toilet paper after you wipe?

    a. Always (**1**)

    b. Sometimes (**2**)

    c. Never (**3**)

3. Before you flush, take a look at the toilet. What color is your poop?

    a. Red (**1**)

    b. Pale yellow, green, or other colors (**2**)

    c. Brown (**3**)

4. After you poop, how often do you feel like the pooping was incomplete?

    a. Always (**1**)

    b. Sometimes (**2**)

c. Never (**3**)

5. How severe is the anal pressure?

a. Extremely—I feel constant pressure and keep going back to the bathroom. (**1**)

b. Somewhat—there's still some stool in me after I poop. (**2**)

c. Not at all—most of my poop comes out during one session. (**3**)

Your Post-Poop Score:

5 to 8	Uh-Oh! 😓
9 to 12	So-So! 😐
13 to 15	Hooray! You Go-Go! 😊 😊 💩

NURSE WONG'S NOTES ON THE POST-POOP

Wiping. Question one ties in with your poop texture and the ease of pooping. If you wipe gently and there's nothing on your toilet paper, then you've really got your poop act together! Unfortunately, this is not the case for most people.

Some of my patients tell me they have to wipe excessively after they poop to feel clean. If you wipe too much, you can irritate your skin, which obviously doesn't feel too good (think butt rash and all kinds of problems). Use a peri bottle, a squeeze bottle with a narrow neck, to spray some water at your bum, or dampen the toilet paper with water and lotion and try to wipe gently. This might help clean off the majority of poop and make picking up any sticky cling-ons easier.

If you feel the need to wipe excessively because there is always brown on your toilet paper or streaks on your underpants, it could mean that your poop is too soft or watery. In this case, you need to add more fiber and cut down your fat intake. Surprisingly, even artificial sugar can make your stool too soft. Try to monitor and adjust your diet for a few weeks and see if your poop texture improves.

Bleeding. The second question should be a no-brainer. Bleeding is not normal, but it can occur without pain or without having anything serious going on. You might have eaten something irritating to your gut, like some whole seeds, tough roughage, or spicy food.

Bright red means the bleeding comes from somewhere close to or at the opening. It could be a hemorrhoid or fissures. If the blood is dark brown like coffee grounds, that means it comes from the higher part of the intestine. In this case, go see a specialist as soon as you can, because it could be something serious.

Color. Your poop color should normally be brown. If yours is a different color (really, any color of the rainbow), it could be due to food dyes, medications, or some underlying health problems. I have made a "Poop Color" video series on my YouTube channel, *Butt Talks TV*. Check that out to see what a particular color might mean and what you could do about it.

Completeness. Question four is not always easy to answer. However, if your poop has enough bulk, and if you sit with the right posture, you should be able to complete your bowel movement.

If your bowel movements feel incomplete, try adding more fiber to your diet to bulk up your stool (certain fruits, vegetables, grains, and fiber supplements) so next time it will come out bigger and move out the leftover poop. If worse comes to worse, you can use a suppository or an enema bottle with the lubricated tip inserted in the anus to rinse out the remaining poop. If these strategies don't work, there may be an underlying condition necessitating you to get checked out by a GI specialist.

Anal Pressure. Question five follows up from number four. The feeling of an incomplete bowel movement can be due to micro-spasms of the butt muscles. Do some deep breathing to relax yourself and your rectal muscles if anal pressure or spasm is still present. You can also try soaking your butt in warm water on a sitz pan or in a bathtub, or lie down to relax your back. If it's inconvenient for you to lie down, try doing some gentle Kegel exercises, where you squeeze and relax your anal muscles as you slowly breathe in and out. These simple tips can be very helpful in alleviating any undue pressure on your anal muscles.

If, after completing all sections of the 3P Questionnaire, you find out you're an "Uh-Oh" person, you are constipated and need help.

A midrange "So-So" score indicates you have moderate pooping issues and may need to make some changes to your diet and lifestyle.

And if you fell into the "Hooray! You Go-Go" category, your pooping process is working amazingly well!

* * *

I hope the poop quiz and 3P Questionnaire helped you gain some insight into the status of your own pooping process. Next, we're going to explore the not-so-pleasant universe of constipation. You might be surprised at how many people are seriously stuck in that tightly bound place, trying to escape so they can one day experience the true power of pooping!

CHAPTER 3

CONSTIPATION AIN'T NO FUN!

*"And therefore, sir, as you desire to live,
a day or two before your laxative, take
just three worms, no under nor above,
because the gods unequal numbers love…
And of ground ivy add a leaf or two. All
which within our yard or garden grow. Eat
these, and be, my lord, of better cheer:
Your father's son was never born to fear."*

—Geoffrey Chaucer,
14th-century English poet and author

ELLA'S STORY: GETTING SHORT-TERM HELP

Ella's mom, Diana, calmly listens to her as she pours her heart out over the phone. When she senses that Ella has unloaded most of her troubles, she tries to put things in perspective so she can say something helpful and supportive. Diana is a retired nurse. She knows that Ella is hurting and likely suffering from some unhealthy habits, so she does her best to empathize with her and make gentle suggestions.

"I'm so glad you were able to share your troubles with me. I know you feel overwhelmed, and I am here to help you any way I can. Are you taking good care of yourself, honey? Are you eating, drinking water, and getting plenty of sleep?"

She waits for a response until she hears Ella speak through muted sobs. "I, I guess I kind of forgot about paying attention to myself because there is so much to do at work to meet all the deadlines, Mom. I either eat on the run or don't eat at all. I drink a lot of black coffee and very little water, and I only sleep four to five hours a night." Ella, sounding like she's gasping for air, continues, "I…just…don't…have time…to do…everything I need…to do…for work, Mom."

Diana runs through some visualization exercises with Ella to help her calm down. Ella pauses for a while before she snaps out of her trance-like state and quietly says, "Thank you, Mom. That really helped. But now I just wish I could take a great big poop, and I can't!"

Since Diana lives close by, she tells Ella to try to relax and that she will be there in about an hour. Ella sits on the pot and tries to poop without success before her mom arrives. When

Ella finally buzzes her mom in, Diana is carrying a large tote bag, ready to go into her Mom's-here-to-care-for-you mode. Like magic, she pulls a scanning thermometer out of her bag, waits for it to calibrate, then holds it to Ella's forehead. The readout indicates that Ella has a low-grade fever. The nurse in Diana then fires off a series of questions about Ella's overall health. Satisfied with her answers, Diana holds up a box containing two enema bottles and comments, "If these don't get you pooping, honey, I don't know what will!"

Sure enough, with her mother's help, Ella takes in the contents of one enema bottle and lies on her left side for ten to fifteen minutes until she feels it taking effect. Like a little kid, she is delighted once she sits on the pot and a liquid poop mixture starts coming out. After going a few more times like this, she is reasonably confident all the enema contents have come out. Diana then assists her with taking a second enema that produces more poop and liquid and helps relieve most of Ella's abdominal pain. Following the release of the second enema, Ella feels giddy and tired. Diana makes sure she drinks two full glasses of water, then tucks her into bed at 7:00 p.m. After twelve straight hours of sleep, Ella wakes up to the warmth of her mother lying by her side. She feels better than she has in months.

Ella calls in sick that morning to get better rested and to spend more time with her mom. As they are chatting, Diana suggests

she get an appointment with Dr. Jackson, a well-known gas-
troenterologist (GI), to assess her digestive system and check
for any complications. Although reticent, Ella finally agrees to
call Dr. Jackson's office and makes an appointment to see
her on the first possible opening, which is three weeks away.

Ella could very well be on track to see an advanced nurse
specialist like me. You'll have to follow her story as it continues
in Chapter 4.

A LITTLE ABOUT ME AND MY PAST POOP PROBLEMS

Many of my patients and friends ask me, "How in the world did you get into this business?" I laugh whenever I hear it, since I know I've taken an unusual departure from traditional nursing. I often respond, "Look, it wasn't my focus in nursing school to specialize in poopatology. I sort of 'fell into it' (the specialty, not the poop) as the need arose in the medical center. It didn't take long for me to realize how prevalent pooping problems are and how important it is for people to have a healthy gut." Along the way, the science and power of pooping captivated me so much that helping people with poop problems became a vital role for me as a nurse. To be honest, poopatology really excites me! So, I found my calling and became a poop missionary, on a mission to help everyone poop better!

Like most bodily functions, the pooping process involves a complex system, but it is also very mechanical. Certain requirements are necessary for the composition of a healthy stool, which you will find more about as you read on. As I mentioned in Chapter 1, we eat our food and never think about what happens to it at the other end. We take our digestive system for granted, thinking that pooping will just happen on its own, and then hope for the best. That is, until we run into unexpected problems with the process that often have messy results.

I thought that way, too, until I ran into my own pooping problems related to some major stressors in my life. The first time was when I was studying for finals in nursing school, just before I was set to graduate. The second was when I was a surgical nurse stuck in the OR for long periods of time, with no bathroom breaks. And the third time was shortly after my son was born. During those tough times, everything related to the regularity of my pooping seemed to turn upside down and backward.

Like Ella, I had constipation, which happens to be one of the most frequently reported poop problems on the planet. Before my constipation developed, pooping just happened, regardless of what I ate or drank. Delivering my son, Julien, required a period of prolonged labor that left me exhausted. I remember quite vividly after his birth that I couldn't even pee on my own, let alone take a poop. It wasn't until a nurse practitioner came to visit me and my son after delivery that I brought up my problems peeing and pooping. She matter-of-factly told me, "You need to RELAX!" After pushing so hard to birth my son, the idea of relaxing to poop took on a whole different meaning. Those problems were big-time wake-up calls that really got my attention and spurred me to eventually become a "butt whisperer," another title affectionately bestowed on me by my coworkers.

LET'S TALK CONSTIPATION

What are the symptoms of constipation? The National Institute of Diabetes and Digestive and Kidney Diseases, or NIDDK (niddk.nih.gov), lists the four main symptoms of constipation as:

- Fewer than three bowel movements per week
- Stools that are hard, dry, or lumpy
- Stools that are difficult to pass
- A feeling that not all stool has passed

Other reported signs and symptoms of constipation include abdominal bloating and pain, the feeling of a blockage in your rectum, and the need for help in stimulating your body to poop, such as massaging the abdomen or using a finger to get the anal muscles working.

Almost all of us experience constipation at some point in our lives. The NIDDK reports that around sixteen out of one hundred adults in the US exhibit symptoms of constipation and about thirty-three out of one hundred adults aged sixty years and older experience those symptoms. Occasional or periodic symptoms of constipation are not a serious concern, but when they become chronic, several red flags may appear to medical professionals.

WHAT CAUSES CONSTIPATION?

In general, constipation happens when your poop moves too slowly through your intricate system of plumbing, or when it can't be expelled from the rectum through your anus, causing the stool to become hard and dry. It's important to understand that constipation is a symptom, not a disease. It's a sign that there is an imbalance or issue with your digestive system. Constipation can happen to you for a variety of reasons, some as simple as too little hydration, not enough dietary fiber, or too many rich foods or sweet desserts. Other reasons may include the overuse of laxatives or enemas that can make your body "forget" how to function on its own. Physical inactivity can be a big contributor to constipation, as movement and gravity stimulate peristalsis. Ignoring the urge to poop and holding it in can lead to constipation. Many medications also contribute to this condition. Other serious causes are listed below.

Blockages of the colon or rectum

- Anal fissures (small tears in anal skin)

- Bowel obstructions

- Colon cancer

- Bowel strictures (narrowing of the colon walls)

- Cancers of the abdomen that press on the walls of the colon

- Cancer of the rectum

- Rectocele, occurring primarily in women, is a bulge of the rectum into the back wall of the vagina

- Rectal prolapse, where the inner lining of the rectum slips down or slides out of the anal opening

Colon and rectal nerve problems (these affect nerves that contract the muscles that move stool through the intestines)

- Autonomic neuropathy—damage to major nerves that control bodily functions

- Multiple sclerosis (MS)

- Parkinson's disease

- Spinal cord injury
- Stroke

Pelvic muscle disorders
- Anismus, or the inability to relax pelvic muscles to facilitate pooping
- Dyssynergia, or pelvic muscles that don't properly coordinate relaxation and contraction
- Weakened pelvic muscles

Previous surgeries
- Colon surgeries that affect muscle and nerve function in the pelvic floor area
- Back surgeries that affect nerve and muscle function of the pelvic floor area
- Corrective surgeries for rectal prolapses

Diseases and conditions that upset the hormonal balance
- Diabetes
- Hyperparathyroidism, or an overactive parathyroid gland
- Pregnancy (it happened to me)
- Hypothyroidism, or an underactive thyroid gland

THE POWER OF *Pooping*

WHAT IS THE PREVALENCE OF CHRONIC CONSTIPATION?

Since occasional symptoms of constipation can often be corrected with small changes in diet and lifestyle, it is not considered a serious issue. However, it becomes a major issue when it morphs into a chronic condition. Let me help you get a clearer overview to see how you may be affected by one of the most frequent poop problems in the US.

There are two types of chronic constipation: irritable bowel syndrome with constipation (IBS-C) and chronic idiopathic constipation (CIC), in which the cause of constipation is unknown. Although everyone experiences constipation at some point in time, it is estimated that over fifty-three million Americans (more frequent in women) suffer from some type of chronic constipation compared to sixty-three million people worldwide, so the incidence is much higher in the US than anywhere else on the planet. According to a 2017 statnews.com article by Warraich, this problem has necessitated millions of visits to clinics annually, as well as 700,000 trips to ERs.[5] Since 1997, the number of hospital admissions for constipation has doubled, and the money spent on laxatives amounts to billions of dollars each year. These statistics

---

5.   Haider J. Warraich, "Beyond Aggravation: Constipation Is an American Epidemic," *STAT*, August 17, 2017, https://www.statnews.com/2017/08/17/constipation-bowels-colon.

clearly indicate that constipation is a very BIG problem in the US. Despite the numbers, it is heartening to know that, if you occasionally suffer from constipation, you are not alone and, in many cases, it can be resolved via diet and lifestyle changes.

Individuals suffering from chronic constipation often have many of the same basic causes and risk factors as those with mild to periodic symptoms, but the symptoms have never been adequately addressed and often continue to worsen.

Some common causes and factors related to chronic constipation are:

- Age and sex—adults sixty-five and older, and women of any age, are more likely to have chronic constipation
- Dehydration
- Diets with low fiber content
- Inactivity/sedentary lifestyle
- Medications such as sedatives, opioids for pain, certain antidepressants, and some meds to lower your blood pressure
- Mental health conditions like depression or eating disorders

Complications of chronic constipation include:

- Swollen anal veins (hemorrhoids). Straining to poop can cause this.

- Torn skin in your anus (anal fissure). Hard turds can cause this.

- Turds that can't be expelled (fecal impaction). Accumulated hardened turds can get stuck in your colon.

- Rectal prolapse, or part of the large intestine stretching and protruding from your anus. Excessive straining to poop can cause this.

As you can readily see, a host of conditions can cause constipation. In the previous chapter, some of the answers that added up to the lowest scores for an Uh-Oh result on the Poop quiz and the 3P Questionnaire had to do with constipation. If you scored in the So-So range, you most likely have periodic bouts of constipation that typically don't require doctor visits.

Another tool I use to help my patients determine their poop health is Nurse Wong's Poop Pictogram on the next page.

NURSE WONG'S POOP PICTOGRAM

1		**Separate hard turds**
2		**Sausage-shaped lumpy turds**
3		**Sausage-shaped turds with surface cracks**
4		**Smooth banana-shaped turds**
5		**Soft chunks with clear cut edges**
6		**Applesauce-like diarrhea**
7		**Liquid diarrhea with no form**

In terms of the shape and texture of your turds, number 1 matches the constipation scenario. Numbers 2 and 3 follow closely behind, as straining is often involved to get those turds out. If you see stools resembling those of numbers 5 to 7, you've gone the other direction into the squishy, poopy world of diarrhea. Number 4 is the ultimate poop that slides out within a few minutes of sitting on the throne with no pushing or straining and features full-figured banana-shaped turds with a smooth texture. Oh, what a relief it is to poop!

BUTTY'S SIDENOTE

Butt Talks TV has made understanding the pooping process easy for you, with the help of many educational videos by Nurse Wong. Scan this QR code to go to the Butt Talks website and check them out:

HOW IS CONSTIPATION DIAGNOSED?

As I mentioned earlier, many different causes of constipation are unseen to the patient or casual observer. Some of them are straightforward, while others are very complex. The complex cases most often cast me in the role of poop detective, amicably interrogating my patients, sifting through previous medical reports, and trying to piece together all the evidence or lack thereof to get to the bottom (pun intended) of their issue(s).

Most of the constipated patients I see have already visited their primary care physician (PCP) or GI, and for the majority of them, the doctor recommended OTC or prescription laxatives. They often come to me when, despite their doctor visits and use of laxatives, they still have issues with constipation, or the laxatives have had the opposite effect—causing loose stools and diarrhea. The first thing I do is go over their history in detail by looking at their responses to the seventeen-page case history forms they have hopefully completed before their appointment.

I often have to explain the meaning of questions on the form and to query my patients extensively to clarify their responses to them. This part can be grueling because sometimes they've only filled out one or two pages of the form and stopped, or worse, they haven't completed anything at all, saying they didn't have time or didn't understand any of the questions. Nevertheless, in my poop detective mode I never skip the history, even if I have to speak to the patient, family member, or interpreter in the simplest of terms to get the most accurate picture of their poop health.

As I mentioned, these patients have previously seen a physician who has performed a general physical assessment, including a digital rectal exam. For you younger readers, in this case "digital" means probing the rectum with the lubricated forefinger of a gloved hand to evaluate the area for any unusual growths such as tumors, cysts, hemorrhoids, or several other possible conditions. Another common in-office procedure performed is an anoscopy, where the doctor inserts an anoscope (a small lighted tube) into your lubricated anus to visually check for anal fissures, hemorrhoids, rectal polyps, and cancer. This is sometimes, but not always, followed by a battery of tests and procedures to diagnose chronic constipation in hopes of determining the cause.

If you have chronic constipation and plan to see a GI or colorectal physician, you should be aware that you may undergo a long list of tests that will help them do the detective work necessary to find out what is causing your problems.

Blood tests. Specifically designed to help your doctor check for systemic bodily conditions like hypothyroidism (low thyroid) and high levels of calcium.

X-ray. X-rays can provide your doctor with the images of your bowels to help him or her determine if you have any blockages or if there's impacted poop throughout your colon.

Rectal exam and sigmoidoscopy. This is an exam of the sigmoid, or lower colon. Your doctor inserts a thin, flexible lighted tube with a camera into your anus to look for obstructions, polyps, blockages, fissures, cancer, and signs of infection in your rectum and sigmoid.

Colonoscopy. This is an exam of the rectum and the entire colon. Your entire colon is examined by the doctor via a flexible tube equipped with a lighted camera. The doctor is looking for many of the same issues as mentioned above, but it allows for a deeper and more detailed look at the full length of the colon. This exam is performed while you are under sedation, so there is typically no pain or discomfort during or afterward.

Anorectal manometry. To assess the anal sphincter muscle function, a doctor, nurse practitioner, or nurse like me inserts a narrow, flexible tube in your anus and rectum, then inflates a small balloon on the end of the tube. This device is then pulled back through the sphincter muscle to allow me or the doctor to measure the way your muscles coordinate to move your bowels. The results are seen on a computer screen.

Balloon expulsion test. This test is an assessment of anal sphincter muscle speed and is typically performed by me, your doctor, a nurse practitioner, or an advanced nurse in conjunction with an anorectal manometry to measure the exact amount of time it takes you to push a water-filled balloon out of your rectum.

Colonic transit study. This procedure assesses how food moves through the colon. It involves swallowing a capsule containing either radiopaque markers, 24 small plastic rings, that designate specific areas or interest on an X-ray or a wireless recording device that records the capsule's progress through your colon over a period of 24 to 48 hours. An alternate form of the procedure involves eating radiocarbon-activated food along with swallowing a capsule containing a small specialized camera that records its progress. Your doctor looks for signs of intestinal muscle dysfunction and how well the food moves through your colon.

Dynamic X-ray defecography. This is an X-ray of the rectum while you're pooping. It is considered the gold standard imaging procedure for capturing issues related to constipation. The doctor inserts soft barium paste into your rectum, which is later passed just like poop. It shows up on the X-rays and can reveal a rectal prolapse or issues with rectal muscles and muscle coordination.

MR defecography. The doctor puts a contrast gel in your rectum. Soon after, you pass the gel while the MRI scanner visualizes and assesses how your defecation muscles are functioning. It can also help diagnose issues related to constipation, such as rectocele or prolapse.

Stool sample. Your doctor may get a stool sample from you if bacterial infection, parasites, tapeworms, or other nasty invaders are suspected of contributing to your constipation.

EMG Recruitment Test. An adjunct test that is often performed concurrently with anorectal manometry, an anal electromyography (EMG) recruitment measures the electrical activity of the anal and rectal muscles (via a small electrode in your rectum) as you relax, squeeze, and gently push as if you were having a BM (bowel movement). This test causes slight discomfort, only takes five minutes to perform, and helps the doctor determine if those all-important muscles are working as they should.

Pudendal Nerve Test. Another test regularly performed in my clinic, although not offered in many facilities, is the pudendal nerve test. The two small pudendal nerves are located at the bottom of the spinal cord. They are critically important for proper functioning of the bowels and bladder as well as the male and female sex organs. (I wasn't kidding when I said *critically important*!) If the cause of your constipation relates to an injury or weakness of the muscles in the anal wall, this test can help determine if the pudendal nerves that stimulate them are functioning properly. The test can also help diagnose fecal incontinence, or lack of control of the bowels. (A very yucky condition!)

For this test, your anus is lubricated and a small probe with an electrode is attached to the practitioner's gloved forefinger and inserted into your rectum. Once the correct position is located, a distinctive wave pattern is seen on the computer screen and soon after, you'll feel a twitching or pulsing sensation from the small electrical current that causes your pelvic floor muscles to contract. The electrode measures and records the time it takes for the responses to occur, in milliseconds. The results help determine if there is damage to the pudendal nerves that contribute to your bowel problems. The test serves to provide supporting evidence to the findings of the primary tests listed above.

HOW IS CONSTIPATION TREATED?

After doing my thorough poop detective work to determine a patient's specific situation, I focus on diet and lifestyle changes and try to steer away from recommending prescription laxatives. The reason I do this is because I see so much overuse of laxatives and so little emphasis on changing daily dietary and lifestyle habits, which are healthier ways of treating constipation. Some of you are using heavy laxatives up to three times a day but not sufficiently hydrating, eating fiber-filled foods, or getting adequate physical exercise.

In reflecting on your average five-to-seven-minute doctor visits, I can't help but see that, for some medical professionals, it is quicker and easier to simply prescribe laxatives and perhaps fiber supplements than to spend more time discussing a daily regimen of healthy poop-producing food and physical activity with you. Don't get me wrong, I love and respect the medical professionals I work with every day, as well as the referring physicians. However, not all of them have the luxury of time and resources to help effect such major life changes. That's where healthcare specialists like me often come into your poop picture.

The physicians who have excellent support staff, such as nurse practitioners (NPs), physician assistants (PAs), or advanced clinical nurses like myself, often perform the initial exams but leave the special testing and counseling to us. Physicians who have minimal help typically order the tests and prescribe laxatives without going into dietary or lifestyle changes, other than perhaps giving you a handout to take home and read.

I would like to believe that most medical support staff, like myself, take the time needed to involve you in the testing process, explain the results, and counsel you on optimal dietary and daily living changes to give you what I call a total "bowel makeover!"

After studying your history, however, I often come to the realization that you have visited multiple physicians and support staff because you are still all bound up; that you are seeing me as a last resort in hopes of avoiding surgery.

For constipation, your bowel makeover starts with increasing your fiber intake to increase the size and weight of your stools, speeding up their movement through your intestines. This involves gradually adding fresh fruit, vegetables, and whole grain cereals and breads to your diet each day. If you add these foods too fast, you may become bloated and gassy (much to the chagrin of your family or friends). When you begin making these important changes, I often recommend the moderate use of fiber supplements in addition to adding fiber-filled foods to your diet. If you're not sure where to begin, I have provided some sample diets in Part 2 so you're not shooting in the dark.

Proper hydration based on your body weight is also critically important to help the waste move more efficiently through your plumbing system. I will share my weight-based hydration formula in Chapter 4, so you know how much water you need to drink each day.

Along with those dietary changes, exercising most days of the week helps stimulate the activity of your intestinal muscles to facilitate more frequent release of those smooth, full-figured turds I mentioned earlier. Whether or not you belong to a gym, it's a good idea to find either a personal trainer or a friend to help you get started on an exercise program that aligns with your health and physical limitations.

I share other important poop habits in counseling, such as paying attention to your urges to poop when they occur and refraining from pushing or straining the muscles that will work involuntarily at the right time, if you let them. Many of you have to learn how to listen to your body's signals and then to act upon them by relaxing and allowing your rectal muscles to do their job: inflate when filled with poop, and deflate when releasing the poop with little to no effort on your part.

LAXATIVES TO LOOSEN YOUR POOP

As I mentioned earlier, literally billions of dollars are spent on both OTC and prescription laxatives each year in this country. Six major types of OTC laxatives are commonly used by patients and/or recommended by medical professionals. These consist of:

OVER-THE-COUNTER LAXATIVES

Laxative Type	How it works	Products
Fiber products	Bulk up your stools so they are softer and easier to pass	Calcium polycarbophil (FiberCon, Equalactin) Methylcellulose (Citrucel) Psyllium (Metamucil, Konsyl)
Stimulants	Act to contract your intestinal muscles	Bisacodyl (Correctol, Dulcolax) Sennosides (Senokot, Ex-Lax, and Perdiem)
Osmotics	Stimulate your colon to increase fluid secretion and facilitate easier bowel movements	Magnesium citrate powder Oral magnesium hydroxide (Phillips' Milk of Magnesia, Dulcolax Milk of Magnesia) Lactulose (Cholac, Constilac) Polyethylene glycol (MiraLAX and GlycoLax)
Lubricants	Enable your poop to more easily move through your colon	Mineral oil
Stool softeners	Moisten your poop by drawing water from your intestines	Docusate sodium (Colace) Docusate calcium (Surfak)
Enemas and suppositories	Hydrate and soften stools using commercial saline solutions or tap water/ soapsuds to produce bowel movements	Fleet enema
Bisacodyl or glycerin	Provide lubrication and stimulation to move the poop out of your rectum	Dulcolax

Meds that draw water into your intestines	Bring water into your intestines to speed up the movement of the poop	Linaclotide (Linzess)
		Lubiprostone (Amitiza)
		Plecanatide (Trulance)
Serotonin 5-hydroxytryptamine 4 receptors	Help move poop through your colon by increasing peristalsis	Prucalopride (Motegrity)
Peripherally acting mu-opioid receptor antagonists (PAMORAs—Thank God for acronyms!)	Reverse the constipating effects of opioids on the intestines for those using opioid pain meds	Naloxegol (Movantik)
		Methylnaltrexone (Relistor)

SUPPLEMENTS FOR CONSTIPATION RELIEF

If you are constipated and trying to transition to a healthier lifestyle but are not quite there yet, there are several natural supplements that, when used properly, may help you with constipation.[6]

Magnesium. This mineral in the form of magnesium citrate, magnesium oxide, and magnesium sulfate can improve symptoms of constipation.

- They must be taken in the recommended dosage to benefit you.

---

6. Jillian Kubala, "10 Supplements That May Help Relieve Constipation," Healthline Media, February 12, 2021, https://www.healthline.com/nutrition/supplements-for-constipation.

- Please be aware that magnesium sulfate can cause GI disturbances such as bloating and diarrhea.

- Health-care providers do not recommend magnesium supplements if you have kidney disease.

Probiotics. Probiotics help support a healthy microbiome, as well as reduce symptoms of constipation. My recommended brand is Jarro-Dophilus, which contains over five billion live bacteria from four strains of *Lactobacillus* and two strains of *Bifidobacterium,* among others. Studies have shown that probiotics can contribute to:

- Better intestinal movement of waste

- Increased stool frequency

- More consistent stools

Fiber. Psyllium fiber, which appeared in the laxative table on page 83, is contained in many commercial products. Along with psyllium, here are some other forms of fiber and their benefits:

- Psyllium is soluble fiber that has high water-holding qualities to help bulk up your stools. I recommend Yerba Prima soluble fiber capsules.

- Inulin, another form of soluble fiber, is primarily taken from chicory root. It is not digested or absorbed by the stomach or small intestine. It helps with the propagation of a special bacteria that is beneficial to the gut. It has also been labeled as a prebiotic, as it feeds the "good guy" bacteria already in your gut.

- Glucomannan is also a water-soluble fiber, taken from elephant yam roots. It is a very viscous fiber that speeds up the digestive system for easier, smoother, bulkier poops.

Carnitine. Derived from an amino acid and found in almost all the cells of the human body, this nutrient is important for energy production. A deficiency may lead to constipation. It may benefit individuals with carnitine deficiency who often have motor and intellectual disabilities. These same individuals may take medications that increase excretion of carnitine from their bodies, so the use of carnitine may help provide constipation relief.

Aloe Vera. A natural remedy from the aloe vera plant, aloe vera come in gel, juice, and powdered form. It can increase colon mucus excretion and act as a laxative. It may be beneficial for those who suffer from constipation related to irritable bowel syndrome (IBS). Consult your health-care professional before using aloe vera supplements and avoid long-term use, which can lead to skin irritation, cramping, diarrhea, and toxic hepatitis.

Senna. An herbal laxative derived from the leaves of the cassia plant, several commercial products contain it. I recommend Super Colon Cleanse by Health Plus, which also includes several other herbs, as well as psyllium. An important caveat with senna is that if it is used at higher than recommended dosages over long periods of time, you may suffer adverse effects.

A recent study referenced by healthline.com indicated the following:[7]

- 1 gram of senna daily improved frequency of stools
- 1 gram of senna improved overall quality of life compared with placebo
- Overall majority of participants reported improvements in constipation

Sujiaonori. An edible Japanese river algae rich in fiber, Sujiaonori may help those with constipation and improve GI function. This product is available from kochi-fresh.com.

Lactitol. A laxative composed of sugar lactose that can increase stool volume and gut motility (movement) to relieve constipation. People who use it typically tolerate it well.

---

7.   Daisuke Morishita et al., "Senna versus Magnesium Oxide for the Treatment of Chronic Constipation: A Randomized, Placebo-Controlled Trial," *The American Journal of Gastroenterology* (US National Library of Medicine), accessed August 19, 2021, https://pubmed.ncbi.nlm.nih.gov/32969946/.

CCH1. Composed of Panax ginseng, ginger, Chinese licorice, Bai Zhu, *Aconitum carmichaelii*, and *Rheum tanguticum,* CCH1 is a formulated Chinese medicine that studies suggest may be effective in treating constipation.

MaZiRenWan (MZRW). This formulation of six Chinese herbs has been indicated to help relieve constipation for over two thousand years. It consists of *Cannabis fructus*, *rhei radix et rhizoma*, *Armeniacae semen amarum*, *Paeoniae radix alba, Magnoliae officinalis cortex,*, and *Aurantii fructus immaturus*.[8]

BIOFEEDBACK AND ELECTRICAL STIMULATION THERAPY (NO, NOT SHOCK THERAPY!)

Training your pelvic muscles via biofeedback therapy is another important way to treat constipation, and it happens to be one of my specialties. I am still amazed at how many people do not know how to relax and tighten their pelvic muscles at the right time to facilitate an easy, positive pooping experience.

---

8. Tao Huang et al., "Chinese Herbal Medicine (MaZiRenWan) Improves Bowel Movement in Functional Constipation through Down-Regulating Oleamide," *Frontiers in Pharmacology*, January 23, 2020, https://www.frontiersin.org/articles/10.3389/fphar.2019.01570/full, https://doi.org/10.3389/fphar.2019.01570.

During biofeedback therapy, I insert a specialized sensor into your anus to measure muscle activity. Then I coach you through exercises to alternate tightening and relaxing your pelvic muscles. My equipment measures your muscle activity as you watch a screen to learn and practice how to use your pelvic floor muscles correctly. It may seem odd that you and others may not know how to properly use the pelvic muscles, but I see this phenomenon on a daily basis. Some of the reasons are because those of you who push and strain to poop may have had a constipating diet growing up or poor potty training, and this was "normal" for you. I have found that biofeedback therapy sessions can help break those unhealthy habits and create a new normal for you.

During the biofeedback sessions, I often introduce the use of electrical stimulation therapy of the pelvic floor muscles to both males and females. This is often employed for those of you who, for whatever reason, have lost control or never learned how to control them properly. This type of therapy, similar to a transcutaneous electrical nerve stimulation (TENS) unit used by physical therapists, involves the placement of a small electrode inside the rectum, and/or the vagina in females, that delivers a painless, light electric current that can be adjusted to different strengths and time intervals.

The electrical stimulation causes the pelvic floor muscles to contract and strengthen, which helps train you to locate, identify, and isolate them in order to gain control for better pooping, whether you are constipated or have fecal incontinence. Besides helping to strengthen these all-important muscles, this kind of stimulation can also teach you how to relax them. Once you've been taught how to use the stimulators, you have the option to purchase your own device and use it for therapy in the privacy of your own home.

KEGEL EXERCISES

Contrary to popular opinion, Kegel exercises are not just for women. They are for men too! Kegel exercises, when done correctly, can strengthen the pelvic floor muscles. Under the guidance of a trained medical practitioner, you can learn to identify and strengthen your pelvic floor muscles in order to learn how to tighten and relax them. These exercises will help you gain greater control of your pooping, whether you are constipated or have fecal incontinence. As an aside, Kegels are also helpful for those who suffer from urinary incontinence.

DON'T GIVE UP THE SHIP

Despite multiple visits to medical specialists, daily use of laxatives, and diet and lifestyle changes, chronic constipation issues can sometimes remain unresolved, which necessitates surgery. This is likely due to structural abnormalities of the colon such as strictures, blockages, or rectoceles. In some cases, part of your colon may need to be removed.

My goal for your pooping problems, barring any serious medical conditions, is to give you all the tools necessary to empower you, without the overuse of laxatives or medications, and, to paraphrase from William Ernest Henley's, "Invictus," to be the captain of your ship, the master of your fate. From the many patients I've seen through the years, I have come to realize that a large percentage of you suffering from chronic constipation can get your life back by learning what and how much to eat and drink, which I'll cover in the next chapter. This, along with gradual lifestyle changes, can facilitate the most incredible, regular, rich pooping experiences ever!

CHAPTER 4

KNOW THY FOOD

"Your body is your temple. You do your body good, your body will do you good."
—Floyd Mayweather Jr., former US professional boxing champion

ELLA'S STORY: AN ONGOING STRUGGLE

After her mother's visit, Ella feels better. Although she is still suffering from constipation, it doesn't seem to be as bad as it was when it reached a crisis point.

Ella returns to work with a new outlook, one of trying to be kinder to her body and mind in order to nourish her spirit. She strives to be more relaxed and to eat regularly, as well as to drink more water and take more breaks that include deep breathing.

The first couple of days back at work seem to go more smoothly for Ella. She starts to notice that she feels a little better and doesn't get so caught up in the workplace drama.

But her feeling of hope soon becomes so overridden by the daily grind that she gets emotional and cries herself to sleep several nights during that first week back. Despite her good intentions, she quickly gets swept up in the pressure cooker of strategic planning, endless deadlines, and long work days. Ella's work environment has resumed its stressful stranglehold on her.

Although Ella tries to change her diet and lifestyle, her mother, who now calls every few days, tells her that this won't happen overnight. Diana encourages Ella to set small, achievable goals, and then start slowly to make them happen. Ella promises her mom she will do her best to make changes, but in the back of her mind she has a foreboding feeling of helplessness. Ella always likes to feel in control of whatever situation she's in. Now she is worried that making big changes to her way of living will cause her to lose control, affect her job performance, and eventually lead to personal failure.

Even though Ella makes some small changes to her diet—drinking less coffee and more water along with eating more fresh vegetables and salad—she continues to eat pizza and pasta for carbohydrate-fueled energy before her evening workouts. She still feels constipated as she is only pooping one or two times a week, so she decides to start using a well-known OTC osmotic laxative twice a day to get her bowels to work more efficiently. This new strategy certainly opens the poop gates, but now she occasionally leaks some poop into her underwear, which is smelly, messy, and embarrassing.

Because of her embarrassing bouts of leaky stools, Ella periodically calls in sick and begins to wallow in self-pity. She pretty much gives up on changing her approach to eating and on using strategies to relax at work. She prays that her upcoming appointment with Dr. Jackson will provide a magical cure for all her poop-plagued conditions.

Dr. Jackson, a warm, caring woman, has seen her share of "Ellas" throughout her long career as a gastroenterologist. Observing her fidgeting in the waiting room, Dr. Jackson can readily see that Ella is wrapped up in a ball of stress and is most likely clueless to the overall implications of her condition.

We'll come back to Ella's story in Chapter 5 to see what happens during and after her visit with Dr. Jackson.

FOOD IN THE 21ST CENTURY—
HOW DID WE GET HERE?

PRESERVATION AND STORAGE

Before I give you the scoop on super-poop, I feel it is my duty to discuss the importance of how the power of knowledge translates to the power of positive pooping in your life. The best way I've found to do this is to talk about the evolution or, should I say, the devolution of food trends in the US and other countries that began in the middle part of the 20th century and continues today.

As a society, we moved away from a more agrarian-centered life to a faster-paced urban and suburban lifestyle in the 20th century. The advent of refrigeration, along with a wide range of new gadgets to make it easier and faster to navigate the kitchen and master the once-tedious chore of cooking, ushered in new types of "convenient," prepackaged, foods.

The golden age of television popularized the TV dinner along with other frozen products like vegetables, fruits, and desserts. Along with television came the seemingly nonstop (loud and often irritating) commercial ads for everything under the sun, which included the ginormous amount of new, packaged, frozen, and "instant" food products, not to mention fast foods that also took off in the 1950s and '60s.

Most of those convenience foods (which are still prevalent today) contained mountains of salt, artificial preservatives, emulsifiers (texture stabilizers), and stabilizers to keep them from going bad and to enhance the texture and flavors so consumers would continue to purchase them. They also contained high amounts of fat, carbohydrates, and various forms of sugar that can wreak havoc on your precious plumbing.

Food preservation and storage is nothing new. Inventive ways of preserving and storing food were already being used a few thousand years ago by the Chinese, Egyptians, Romans, Greeks, and Sumerians. Food in ancient times—including meat, vegetables, and fruits—was dried, preserved using salt and sugar, then stored in well-sealed clay jars. Drying foods worked well because fungi and bacteria need moisture to propagate. The salt and sugar produced an environment with high osmotic pressure that denied bacteria the moisture needed to live. Besides the use of salt and sugar to preserve meat and fish, the East Indian and Chinese civilizations utilized spices for preserving foods. They learned to pickle and preserve vegetables using salt, vinegar, lemon juice, or oil of mustard.

Despite these early successful methods of food preservation, it wasn't until the early 19th century that chemists and other scientists understood that bacterial growth was the main cause of spoiled food. The need for new and more sophisticated technology for food preservation was necessitated by the military during the Napoleonic Wars. What was this breakthrough technology? Believe it or not, it was the tin can, which combined heat sterilization with airtight seals.

Early versions of the tin can were made with lead-alloy seals that corroded from the acid in certain food and could be toxic as well. Moving into the late 1950s and '60s, cans were man-

THE POWER OF **Pooping**

ufactured with plastic linings made out of bisphenol A (BPA), which, according to packagingdigest.com, even in trace amounts may cause reproductive, neurological, and immune system problems; heart disease; and type 2 diabetes (which, can affect the digestive system).[9] Although banned by several European countries, BPA has not been banned by the FDA in the US.

Despite the lack of a ban, these health-related discoveries have led the majority of US companies to remove BPA from can linings, replacing it with acrylic and polyester materials that have been extensively tested and cleared by regulatory agencies prior to going on the market. In addition to can liners, many plastic products containing BPA have been found to leach minute amounts of the chemical into the drinks and foods they contain. This has resulted in the removal of many such products from the market. If you're concerned about your overall health, please look for BPA-free containers.

Why am I going into such detail about food preservation and storage? The answer is simple: everything we eat goes through our exquisite network of plumbing, turns into waste, and comes out as poop! It's important to know how what we put into our bodies can affect our overall health. So, in my mind, it's all poop-related!

9. Lisa McTigue Pierce, "BPA Found in Canned Foods Marketed to Kids," *Packaging Digest*, March 11, 2015, https://www.packagingdigest.com/decorative-materials/bpa-found-canned-foods-marketed-kids.

THE EFFECTS OF ARTIFICIAL ADDITIVES

According to sciencemuseum.org.uk, food additives saw a dramatic increase in use during the Industrial Age in the late 1700s to the early 1800s, when certain cheeses and sweets were colored with either red lead or green copper arsenite, both of which are toxic to humans.[10] Chemists continued to create additives and preservatives in the form of thickeners, emulsifiers, and flavor enhancers for many decades. As I mentioned earlier, the widespread use of frozen foods (TV dinners) in the US exploded in the 1950s and '60s, and they were and still are often loaded with high levels of preservatives. TV dinners currently account for around a trillion dollars in sales each year.

It wasn't until well into the 20th century that concerns started growing over the potential toxicity and carcinogenic (cancer-causing) properties of additives. This was due to the development and use of analytic chemistry, which made it easier to detect and measure the properties of food additives.

Preservatives can be natural or artificial. They are not only added to all types of processed foods, but also to cosmetic and pharmaceutical products as well. There are so many different preservatives in products we use every day, from

---

10. "Food: A Chemical History," Science Museum, November 27, 2019, https://www.sciencemuseum.org.uk/objects-and-stories/chemistry/food-chemical-history.

frozen dinners to toothpaste to nasal spray, that I can only zero in on the ones in food that research has found may be hazardous to your health.

Colorectal cancer is the third most common type of cancer that affects both men and women in the US. While the jury is still out, information from nwmedicalspecialties.com reports that extensive research on mice suggests that colorectal cancer may be related to additives called emulsifiers presented in a plethora of processed foods.[11] Researchers have discovered that the consumption of foods with emulsifiers dramatically changed the microbiome, causing significant inflammation and cell death in the digestive tract of otherwise healthy mice. The inflammatory disruptions seen in the intestines of mice may also promote the growth of tumors in the gut. These changes to the microbiome may be risk factors in humans for IBS, which includes Crohn's disease, affecting both the small and large intestines. As mentioned previously, IBS may include constipation (IBS-C), while gut inflammation from Crohn's disease most often causes diarrhea, abdominal pain, and blood in your poop.

A review of the potentially harmful effects of commonly used artificial preservatives listed fifteen that have deleterious health

---

11   Northwest Medical Specialties, "Are Food Additives Linked to Colon Cancer?" Northwest Medical Specialties, March 31, 2017, https://www.nw medicalspecialties.com/blogs/colon-cancer/are-food-additives-linked-to-colon-cancer.

effects on children and adults ranging from hypersensitivity to asthma and different forms of cancer.[12] High on the list for cancer were nitrites and nitrates, often found in processed meats. In fact, a 2020 research review found a significant link between sodium nitrate in certain processed meats to cancer in both the small and large intestine, as well as the rectum.[13]

In addition to a long list of preservatives that can pose potential health risks to humans, certain artificial sweeteners, particularly in the form of sugar alcohols, are culprits as well. Sugar alcohols with names ending in "itol," such as erythritol, mannitol, sorbitol, and xylitol can cause diarrhea in diabetics as well as "normal folks." I find this to be rather ironic for diabetics, since they often opt to consume products with artificial sweeteners.

12. S. P. Anand and N. Sati,"Artificial Preservatives and Their Harmful Effects: Looking Toward Nature for Safer Alternatives," *International Journal of Pharmaceutical Sciences and Research* 12, no. 9 (June 21, 2013): 2496–501.

13. William Crowe, Christopher Elliot, and Brian Green, "A Review of the In Vivo Evidence Investigating the Role of Nitrite Exposure from Processed Meat Consumption in the Development of Colorectal Cancer," *Nutrients* 11, no. 11 (2019). https://doi.org/10.3390/nu1112673.

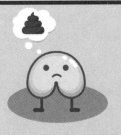

BUTTY'S SIDENOTE

Gut problems are much more common if you are diabetic. A 2018 study referred to by badgut.org revealed that type 1 diabetics reported many more GI issues such as constipation, bloating, abdominal pain, excessive gas, and diarrhea than folks without diabetes.[14] Constipation and diarrhea were twice as likely to occur in those with diabetes than those without it.

WHAT ARE EMPTY-CALORIE FOODS?

Much of what we call "modern" foods and drinks today are full of empty calories. Empty calories come from foods and drinks that have minimal nutritional value. These are mainly items containing a significant amount of added solid fats, processed oils, and sugars. A dietary calorie, by the way, is

---

14. John S. Leeds et al., "Lower Gastrointestinal Symptoms Are Associated with Worse Glycemic Control and Quality of Life in Type 1 Diabetes Mellitus," *BMJ Open Diabetes Research & Care* 6, no. 1 (May 29, 2018).

a unit used to measure the energy value of foods. Here's a partial list of empty-calorie foods so you have a good idea of what I'm talking about.

- Fast foods such as burgers, wraps, pizza, french fries, and more

- Processed oils such as soybean and canola

- Condiments like ketchup and barbecue sauce

- Carbohydrate-based white breads, buns, biscuits, and more

- Sugary liquids, including soda, energy drinks, and fruit juice

- Carbohydrate-based desserts like cookies, cakes, donuts, and more

- Candy bars, hard and soft candies, and chocolates

- Some meats, including hot dogs, bacon, and sausages

- Some full-fat products like butter, ice cream, and shortening

- Alcohol

Okay, so what's the big deal with empty-calorie foods? You may remember back in Chapter 1, when I emphasized that the main purpose of your wonderful plumbing network is to transform the food you put in your body into rich nutrients that provide you with energy, cell repair, and growth. If you eat a lot of empty-calorie foods, where do the nutrients come from to keep your body running smoothly?

Regularly consuming large amounts of empty-calorie food can contribute to weight gain, obesity, and lack of energy. And you may suffer deficiencies of essential vitamins, minerals, protein, fiber, and fatty acids. You might also develop chronic health issues like heart disease, diabetes, and a host of other conditions. When frequently consumed, most of these foods can cause constipation, bloating, and gut inflammation, as well as pose a higher risk for colon cancer. What's really scary to me is that a 2010 study sponsored by the National Institutes of Health found that children and adolescents obtained close to 40 percent of their total calories from empty-calorie foods.[15]

Evidence shows that dietary behaviors tend to stay constant over time, and poor eating habits established in childhood tend to persist through adulthood.[16] A poor diet contributes to the development of four of the nation's ten leading causes of death: coronary heart disease, stroke, diabetes, and certain types of cancer. Other detrimental conditions associated with diet are hypertension, obesity, osteoporosis, and poor

15. "Where Kids Get Their Empty Calories," National Institutes of Health (US Department of Health and Human Services), September 7, 2017, https://newsinhealth.nih.gov/2010/12/where-kids-get-their-empty-calories.

16. "Guidelines for School Health Programs to Promote Lifelong Healthy Eating," Centers for Disease Control and Prevention, June 14, 1996, https://www.cdc.gov/mmwr/preview/mmwrhtml/00042446.htm.

oral health. Over the last decade the number of overweight children and adults has increased significantly. Eating disorders and unsafe weight-loss methods have become more prevalent as well.

I hope I haven't scared the wits out of you by highlighting many of the foods and drinks you shouldn't consume on a daily basis, as well the disease risks to children and adults.

On a positive pooping note, let's find out what foods and drinks are healthier alternatives to the processed and sugary ones and, most importantly, which will help you produce the best smooth, full-figured, banana-shaped super-poops!

STAY HYDRATED!

Do you remember how you used to run around playing with your friends in the summers when you were a kid, and how you could drink, and drink, and drink water from the hose or tap when you got tired out? Depending on your age now, you probably don't drink nearly as much water as you did back then. As we age, our thirst censors become less sensitive to our body's need for hydration, so we tend to drink less water than we need. Exactly how much water should we drink to stay well-hydrated? Here is a simple formula and some tips I use that can serve you well.

THE POWER OF **Pooping**

HYDRATION HELPS AND HABITS

Simply divide your body weight in pounds by 2.2.
The result is how many fluid ounces of water you should drink each day.

$$\frac{\textbf{Body weight in pounds}}{\textbf{2.2}} = \begin{array}{c}\textbf{Fluid ounces of water}\\\textbf{to drink every day}\end{array}$$

Example: If you weigh 160 pounds, you'll need roughly 73 fluid ounces of water, or approximately 9 cups per day.

$$\frac{\textbf{160 pounds}}{\textbf{2.2}} = \begin{array}{c}\textbf{73 Fluid ounces of water}\\\textbf{to drink every day}\end{array}$$

If you follow the metric system, your weight in kilograms is equal to the amount of fluid ounces you'll need to drink per day.

$$\begin{array}{c}\textbf{Body weight}\\\textbf{in kilograms}\end{array} = \begin{array}{c}\textbf{Fluid ounces of water to}\\\textbf{drink every day}\end{array}$$

Example: If you weigh 72 kilograms, you'll need 72 fluid ounces of water per day, which is approximately 9 cups.

$$\textbf{72 kilograms} = \begin{array}{c}\textbf{72 Fluid ounces of water}\\\textbf{to drink every day}\end{array}$$

People who are more active generally need to drink 2 more cups of water per day (approximately 16 fluid ounces or .47 liters more).

Create simple habits to help yourself drink a steady amount of water throughout the day.

Drink water during your meals.

Purchase a reusable water bottle with time markers if that will help remind you to drink your water.

Healthy Hydrating Liquids	Limit your intake of these drinks
Smoothies (with fresh or frozen fruits)	Soda
Homemade soups (not canned)	Coffee
Herbal teas (caffeine-free)	Caffeinated teas
Juices (vegetable and fruit, in moderation)	Alcohol
Milk (cow, goat, almond, soy, and oat); be mindful of allergies and lactose intolerance.	

FIBER, FIBER, AND MORE FIBER!

For those of you with chronic constipation primarily attributed to diet and lifestyle, eating food with good dietary fiber is your best medicine. When I refer to dietary fiber, I mean the parts of plants and carbohydrates you eat but cannot digest. Yes, you heard me right, your body cannot digest them. Fiber is found in all plant foods, including vegetables, fruits, grains, nuts, seeds, and legumes (beans). Another form of fiber, called "chitin," is found in the shells of crustaceans like lobster, shrimp, and crab.

There are two types of fiber: one that is soluble in water and one that is insoluble. Water-soluble fiber slows your digestion to help you absorb those precious nutrients from your food. Insoluble fiber helps bulk up your poop by drawing water into it, which helps your poop move more quickly through your gut and out your butt. Plants typically consist of both types of fiber. Foods with high levels of soluble fiber include oats, oat bran, rice bran, barley, dried beans, apples, strawberries, citrus fruits, potatoes, and peas. Foods with high amounts of insoluble fiber include fruit and vegetable skins, seeds, whole grains, cereals, and wheat bran.

According to webmd.com, the best type of fiber to help with your constipation comes from whole grain breads, cereals, and pastas.[17] Wheat bran cereal can be quite effective as a natural laxative.

The fiber in legumes and citrus fruits provides stimulation for the growth of healthy colonic flora, or the good gut guys I mentioned in Chapter 1. This helps increase the weight of your stools, as well as the amount of good guy bacteria in them.

---

17. Jeanie Lerche Davis, "Top 10 Sources of Fiber," WebMD, October 7, 2005, https://www.webmd.com/diet/features/top-10-sources-of-fiber.

The chitin from shellfish is a great source of insoluble fiber that also provides probiotic components to your gut flora. Some derivatives of chitin have also been found to possess antioxidant properties.[18]

Here are some simple ideas from my YouTube channel, *Butt Talks TV,* for getting your daily dietary fiber.

Daily Fresh Fruits and Vegetables. They give you plenty of fiber to keep your stools soft and stimulate your gut for those dreamy poops. Think of them as the Three S's for smoothies, salads, and soups. (See my recipes in Chapter 9.)

Smoothies. Made with a combination of fruits, veggies, and protein powder, smoothies are a great way to get your fiber and protein with minimal effort. I have a smoothie each morning to start my day.

Salads. A creative and tasteful way to eat plenty of vegetables, salads can be colorful like a rainbow with (preferably certified organic) veggies such as these:

- Leafy greens—romaine lettuce, spinach, kale
- Beets
- Carrots

18. Kaylyn Cade, "What Is Chitin and Why Is It So Cool?" Exo, July 12, 2019, https://exoprotein.com/blogs/blog/what-is-chitin?_pos=1&_sid=c03a6efb7&_ss=r.

- Peppers of all colors

- Avocados

- Any other vegetables you love!

Soups. Soups are another great way to eat plenty of vegetables. Use vegetable or meat broth as a base. Add meat or go meatless. Some veggies to add include the following:

- Sautéed onions

- Carrots

- Celery

- Potatoes (in moderation)

- All types of legumes

Additional Fiber. Don't forget to eat other sources of fiber, such as the following examples:

- Whole grain breads, cereals, and pastas made from

  - Wheat

  - Barley

  - Rye

- Gluten-free grains

  - Amaranth

  - Brown rice

- Farro
- Quinoa
- Oatmeal
- Flaxseed meal

- Root vegetables
  - Carrots
  - Celery
  - Parsnips
  - Potatoes

- Fruits
  - Oranges (all types)
  - Grapefruits
  - Apples
  - Blueberries
  - Prunes
  - Kiwis

Nuts and Seeds. The top ten nuts and seeds from the highest to lowest in fiber are listed below:[19]

---

19. Daisy Whitbread, "Top 10 Nuts and Seeds Highest in Fiber," My Food Data, July 28, 2021, https://www.myfooddata.com/articles/nuts-seeds-high-in-fiber.php.

THE POWER OF *Pooping*

- Seeds

  - Chia

  - Flax

  - Pumpkin and squash

  - Dried coconut

  - Sesame

- Nuts

  - Almonds

  - Pine nuts

  - Pistachios

  - Hazelnuts

  - Pecans

DAILY FIBER RECOMMENDATIONS

On average, most Americans get around 15 grams of fiber daily, which, according to the American Dietetic Association, is much less than what we need. If you're an adult male, your goal should be to eat at least 38 grams of fiber daily. If you're an adult female fifty or younger, you should shoot for 36 grams or more daily. Females who are fifty-one or older should aim to eat at least 21 grams.

BUTTY'S SIDENOTE—AMUSING COMMENTS ABOUT FIBER

Quite often, after I counsel a patient on changing their diet to include more fiber, I hear some interesting comments such as "Fiber? I get my fiber from one apple a day because it keeps the doctor away!" or "I don't have enough money to buy fresh fruits and vegetables. It's quicker and cheaper to go to McDonald's to get my fiber from the bun and lettuce in my Big Mac." This is an example of how some people are simply uninformed about the fiber content in the foods they eat and the amount required each day.

When I was a kid, my grandmother used to eat pitted prunes to keep her regular. I really didn't understand why she ate them or what they did for her (I didn't like them as a kid) until I got older. Prunes are indeed a natural laxative. Just 1 cup of uncooked pitted prunes contains 12 grams of fiber, both soluble and insoluble.

It's always best to get your fiber from food. If for some reason you can't get enough fiber from eating fruits, veggies, and whole grains, then try taking one or two capsules of psyllium powder each day with plenty of water to help you out.

WHAT OTHER HEALTHY FOODS SHOULD I EAT?

To stay healthy and hydrated and consume the fiber you need each day, let's not forget the importance of healthy protein and fatty acids in your diet. Along with your vegetables, which should be the star of your plate, eat plenty of shellfish, fish, and lean meats. The American Heart Association (AHA) recommends that you eat up to 8 ounces of nonfried fish (particularly oily fish like tuna, salmon, mackerel, etc., high in healthy omega-3 fatty acids) each week split into 3.5 to 4 ounces per serving. The AHA also suggests eating no more than 5.5 ounces of nonfried cooked shellfish like shrimp, crab, or lobster, skinless poultry like chicken or turkey, or lean cuts of meat (beef, pork, lamb) each day. Red meats contain saturated (bad) fats that can raise your cholesterol, potentially leading to heart disease. If some of you have trouble digesting meats or just want a break from them, then try eating beans, peas, lentils, or tofu, which are good protein substitutes for meat that you can enjoy in soups, entrees, and salads.

WHAT ABOUT SUGAR?

Soda, sports drinks, and energy drinks add up to more than a third of our daily sugar intake.[20] Sugar, in its many forms, has also been a not-so-secret ingredient in many processed foods for years. If you read the labels on frozen, packaged, or canned foods, you will often see high-fructose corn syrup, corn sweetener, lactose, malt syrup, dextrose, and many other iterations of sugar listed in the ingredients of a wide range of products. Too much added sugar, along with many other additives in processed foods and drinks, contributes to obesity, heart disease, and diabetes.

The AHA recommends women keep to under 100 calories, or 24 grams (about 6 teaspoons) of added sugar per day and men to under 150 calories, or 36 grams (9 teaspoons) each day. It's much harder to keep track of your sugar intake if you eat a number of processed foods. The best rule of thumb is to avoid or seriously limit your consumption of processed foods, sugary drinks, and all types of candy.

---

20 Julie Corliss, "Eating Too Much Added Sugar Increases the Risk of Dying with Heart Disease," Harvard Health, February 6, 2014, https://www.health.harvard.edu/blog/eating-too-much-added-sugar-increases-the-risk-of-dying-with-heart-disease-201402067021.

ARE CARBOHYDRATES BAD FOR YOU?

Carbohydrates have gotten a bad reputation over the years from proponents of low-carb diets. However, carbohydrates, which are converted to glucose (sugar) during digestion, are an important source of fuel and essential nutrients to keep your body healthy. This fuel is particularly important to brain health.

There are two types of carbohydrates:

1. Simple carbs found in sugars, such as table sugar, honey, sodas, fruit, fruit juice, and dairy products

2. Complex carbs composed of long chains of glucose molecules from breads, pasta, crackers, and rice, as well as from starchy vegetables like corn, peas, potatoes, winter squash, and butternut squash

Complex carbs can further be broken down into refined and whole grain carbohydrates

When carbohydrates turn into glucose, this raises our blood sugar. Some carbs do this faster than others. Controlling our blood glucose is critical for weight management, as well as for diabetes. It's important for you to eat *carbohydrates that contain plenty of fiber*, such as broccoli, beans, apples with the skin (and many more of the foods I listed earlier), along with 100 percent whole grain breads, because they help release glucose more slowly into your bloodstream.

Refined carbs found in white bread, white rice, and white pasta have had the fiber and nutrients removed, so the glucose they produce gets into your bloodstream much faster, which can cause spikes in your blood sugar. With high consumption of refined carbohydrates, the risk for developing diabetes (with associated digestive issues like IBS-C) is much higher.

Please know that the complex, fiber-filled carbohydrates I mentioned above provide important fuel and nutrients to your body. However, it's important to remember to eat them in moderation (about one quarter of your plate) and to avoid the simple carbs in sugary drinks, refined white flour grain products, and processed foods.

Get into the habit of reading labels so you know exactly what ingredients are in the foods and drinks you opt to purchase. Try to stay on a regular meal schedule each day to maintain a healthy rhythm for your digestive system. And I'll say it one more time: try to avoid or limit your intake of empty-calorie foods, drinks, sweets, and processed foods, if possible.

According to health.gov, almost half of American adults (117 million people) have one or more preventable chronic diseases, many of which are correlated with poor diet and physical inactivity.[21] Over two-thirds of adults and almost one-third of children are overweight or obese. The medical costs related to obesity were estimated to be around $147 billion in 2008. The medical costs associated with diagnosed diabetes were estimated to be around $245 billion in 2012, which included $69 billion in lower work productivity.[22]

WHAT IS A RECOMMENDED HEALTHY DIET?

According to *2020–2025 Dietary Guidelines for Americans* (downloadable from health.gov), the recommended levels of daily calorie intake vary with age, sex, and level of physical activity. For example, a twenty-five-year-old female who is moderately active should consume about 2,200 calories per day, while a male of the same age and activity level should consume around 2,800 calories daily. Looking at a fifty-year-old female with a moderate activity level, the caloric intake should be around 2,000, and a male of the same age and level of activity should consume about 2,400. In addition,

21. US Department of Health and Human Services and US Department of Agriculture, *2015–2020 Dietary Guidelines for Americans*, 8th ed., December 2015, accessed August 22, 2021, https://health.gov/our-work/food-nutrition/previous-dietary-guidelines/2015.
22. Economic Costs of Diabetes in the U.S. in 2012. Diabetes Care 2013;36:1033-1046," *Diabetes Care* 36, no. 6 (2013): 1797–97, https://doi.org/10.2337/dc13-er06.

these guidelines recommend that you consume less than 10 percent of daily calories from added sugars, less than 10 percent of daily calories from saturated fats, and less than 2,300 milligrams of sodium per day.

A simple way to exemplify a healthy diet is via myplate.gov, created by former First Lady Michelle Obama and former Agriculture Secretary Tom Vilsack. MyPlate is organized into four sections of approximately 30 percent veggies, 30 percent grains, 20 percent fruits, and 20 percent protein, with a smaller amount of dairy on the side.

This simple graphic will help you visualize what I'm referring to.

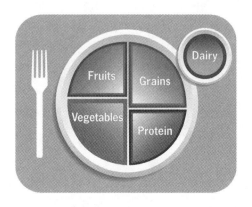

VITAMINS AND MINERALS

No matter how healthy our diets, most of us don't get enough of our vitamins and minerals from food these days. Our bodies

THE POWER OF *Pooping*

run on over 30 vitamins, minerals, and enzymes, nutrients that are critical to the energy we need to live. Taken with meals, high-quality multivitamin and mineral supplements with good bioavailability (the percentage of supplement that reaches the bloodstream) are essential to our survival. Don't forget to read the labels on supplements, as some have many fillers.

When you are ready to commit to making the transition to a healthier diet with plenty of fiber-filled fruits and vegetables, along with whole grains, nuts, seeds, and sources of good protein, flip to the second section of this book. It is a veritable gold mine of weekly meal plans, with recipes for the Three S's, as well as sample menus to get you started on the road to super-poop! Trust me, your gut and your butt will thank you!

CHAPTER 5

TOOLS FOR THE PERFECT POOPING PROTOCOL

"Sometimes all you need to feel better about life is a good poop."

—someecards.com

ELLA'S STORY: GETTING TO THE "BOTTOM" OF THINGS

On a sunny Friday afternoon, Ella is anxiously sitting in Dr. Jackson's waiting room after filling out the necessary paperwork, including a lengthy health history form. She is hoping they call her name soon, before she changes her mind and bolts to the door for a quick escape. Just as that thought passes through her head, she is called to follow the nurse into the clinic.

After the nurse weighs her and takes her vitals, Ella is escorted to an exam room, where she impatiently waits another twenty minutes before Dr. Jackson finally appears and cheerfully greets her. Dr. Jackson quietly reads through the health history form, then speaks to Ella in a soft, gentle voice as she looks her directly in the eyes. Her warm, caring nature immediately begins to put Ella at ease.

After gently probing Ella to elaborate on some of her specific issues with constipation, the stressors of her job, and what she's doing to deal with her condition, Dr. Jackson performs a physical examination. One part of the exam is an anoscopy, during which Dr. Jackson puts a small lighted tube in Ella's anus and takes a quick peek inside her rectum. The final component of the evaluation is a digital exam with her lubricated and gloved right forefinger to check the anatomy of Ella's rectum. While she is feeling for anything unusual, Dr. Jackson briefly hesitates, closes her eyes, checks a specific area again, then finishes the exam. Ella, sensing something is amiss, asks the doctor what's wrong. Dr. Jackson, not wanting to alarm Ella, says, "I'm not exactly sure yet, Ella. I need to order an X-ray defecography of your rectum and have some tests performed on the muscles down there before I can give you a definitive answer."

"The X-ray defecographies are only performed at the Regional Medical Center. I also want to refer you to Dr. Sloan, an excel-

lent colorectal physician I've consulted with for a long time. His clinic is at the Regional Medical Center, so he can get the X-ray results by the next day. His clinic is also equipped to do all the other necessary tests. Is that okay with you?"

Ella, unsure of how to respond, pauses, then softly says, "I guess, I mean, of course that's okay with me, Dr. Jackson. Even though we've just met, I trust you to know what to do to figure out how to help me. Thank you so much."

Dr. Jackson replies, "You're welcome. Now try not to worry Ella. I'll do my best to get the referral completed and the tests ordered as soon as possible." Before Dr. Jackson leaves the room, she asks Ella to cut her laxative use in half, then asks her to follow some simple steps from a handout she gives her. The handout provides tips on how to better hydrate, eat more fiber, get more sleep, and exercise on a daily basis. Ella nods her head, thanks Dr. Jackson again, then finds her way out.

Diana comes to spend the weekend with Ella. Although not the prying type, as a mother she's naturally curious if Ella's appointment with Dr. Jackson shed any light on her problem, so she asks her how it went. Ella takes a few moments before she replies. "Mom, I really like Dr. Jackson. I can tell she cares deeply about her patients. Her warm, gentle nature made me feel very comfortable. She didn't rush the visit and really listened to me. I'm worried though, because she found some-

thing in my rectum that warranted a referral to Dr. Sloan, and she ordered a special X-ray along with several other tests."

Diana probed Ella a little more and found out that Dr. Jackson didn't want to say what she had found or maybe just didn't know for sure. Diana was also familiar with Dr. Sloan and knew that her daughter would be in good hands with him and his top-notch staff. Spending the weekend with Diana gave Ella a safe, warm feeling inside as they chatted away, took walks, shopped, ate fresh salads, and cooked healthy, vegetable-filled meals.

Ella returns to work the following Monday morning. She makes it a point to focus on changing her bad habits. After a solid night's sleep, she has a full glass of water, one cup of fresh coffee, some whole grain wheat toast, and fresh fruit to start the morning. At work she does her best to drink plenty of water and take regular breaks, during which she noshes on more fruit, almonds, and sunflower seeds. For lunch, Ella invites Sandy, her coworker and friend, to join her at a nice downtown restaurant that features a fresh salad bar. Sandy is the bubbly type, always upbeat and positive, which keeps Ella in a good mood.

The rest of her day goes fairly smoothly. When Ella feels the stress brewing like a black cloud moving in to envelop her, she remembers to stop and take several deep breaths, just as her mother taught her. This helps a lot but, although she feels better, Ella can't stop her thoughts from drifting back to the look on Dr. Jackson's face when she found something unusual during the digital rectal exam.

While she continues to work on making gradual changes for the better, Ella still feels constipated, even though she pooped out a few skinny turds with a funny hook on one end twice in the last three days. She cut her laxative use in half as Dr. Jackson recommended, but she is having sensations that more poop is built up inside her rectum and she has to go. Despite her efforts at pushing and straining, nothing comes out.

The next day Ella receives two phone calls: one from the medical center and the other from Dr. Sloan's office. The scheduler for the X-ray defecography has an opening Wednesday, the very next day, at 11:00 a.m., while Dr. Sloan's receptionist has just had a cancellation, so she offers her an appointment on Thursday at 1:00 p.m. Ella feels as if the stars are aligning perfectly for both appointments. She decides that it's best to find out what's going on and have it taken care of as soon as possible, so she books both appointments. We'll come back to Ella's story in Chapter 6.

HOW TO PROPERLY POOP

You'd be surprised at how many patients I've seen who, like Ella, push, strain, and completely dread every moment of pooping or attempting to poop. Despite the changes in diet and lifestyle needed to help resolve constipation, I think it's important to discuss some tools for better pooping, starting with how to poop properly. Now you might say to yourself, "This is ridiculous, I already know how to poop the right way! I've been pooping fine my whole life." If you dread your poop time on the toilet, however, you may be missing out on the glorious experience it could be with a little power of pooping knowledge and experience. Here are some simple tips for a perfect pooping experience:

THE URGE

If you feel the urge, don't wait! Poop as soon as possible. Waiting too long is not good for you.

THE SEARCH

Find a comfortable place to poop. If in public, check multiple bathroom stalls for the best selection. Here's what you should avoid:

- Wobbly toilet seats
- Stalls with faulty or missing door locks

- Dirty toilet seats
- Little or no toilet paper

PUBLIC POOPING PROTOCOL, OR THE THREE P'S

Pre-Poop. Now that you've found your toilet seat, be sure to wipe it down with TP. If you carry hand sanitizer or a cleaning wipe, that is a bonus. Before you begin, here are some poop tips:

- Once you've wiped the toilet seat, put paper in the middle of the toilet bowl to prevent water from splashing back on your butt when you poop.
- If it's an automatic flush toilet, drape a few sheets of TP over the sensor to avoid surprise flushes

Remember, being on the toilet should be a peaceful experience, not one with unpleasant poopy water splashing on your butt!

Poop. Now it's time to relax on the toilet. One technique I use is a slow breathing pattern:

- Hold a piece of tissue in front of your mouth.
- Blow on it gently enough so the tissue paper moves slightly back and forth.

- Be sure to do this three times while relaxing your butt muscles.

- You should feel your pelvic muscles drop slightly.

Ideally, you should not push at all. However, if you do, try not to push too hard or too long. Allow time for your butt muscles to relax between pushes. Pushing can cause many butt-related problems, such as hemorrhoids and rectal pain, and can block your stool from coming out completely.

One way to release the stool is through a gentle Kegel, where you slightly contract your anal muscles inward then exhale to release. Another helpful tool is proper pooping posture. Be sure to sit in a position where your poop comes out quickly and easily. There is not a one size-fits-all position.

- Sit upright while slightly leaning forward at a 35-degree angle. It may be helpful to put your feet on a small bench or stool to get the best poop angle. Or, try slightly leaning backward.

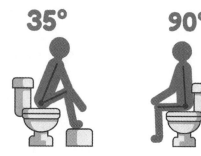

- Place your hands on your knees or wherever comfortable.

- Whether you're male or female, pull your slacks down to your ankles so you can widen your legs with your knees apart.

- Finally, plant your feet flat on the ground or slightly raise your heels while placing your weight on the balls of your feet.

Exceptions to these rules depend on

- Your height
- Toilet height
- Your butt size

Post-Poop. Now we've reached the final stage of pooping. Be sure to clean well, as this prevents underwear stains, irritation, and potential infection. Here are a few helpful tips to try when wiping:

- When wiping, sitting or standing doesn't matter as long as you can reach your butt.

- It's best to reach behind you, wiping from front to back. This ensures the poop is moving away from your genitals to help prevent infections.

- Be sure not to wipe too hard, as this can cause irritation.

- Adding a pea-sized dot of fragrance-free face skin cream or water onto the paper can further help clean your butt.

- Don't fill the toilet up with too much toilet paper, as this can clog it.

- You can also use biodegradable body wipes, but be sure to throw them into the garbage rather than flushing them.

- Whether you're at home or traveling, a more lasting butt cleanse would be to wash it with water. This can include using a bidet or a handheld wet nap, or taking a bath or shower while paying special attention to your bottom.

- If you have hemorrhoids, irritated butt skin, or itchiness, use one or more of the many products available to help soothe this sensitive area. Depending on your specific problem, products such as Calmoseptine, Desitin Daily Defense, witch hazel extract (follow directions on the bottle), and tea tree essential oil (mix 2 drops with 12 drops of olive, coconut, or almond oil to dilute, then put 3 to 4 drops on a cotton ball and apply to the skin) may provide relief.

If possible, close the toilet lid when flushing to reduce the spread of germs. (See Butty's Sidenote on page 130.)

Finally, be sure to wash your hands with soap and water. If that's not available, use hand sanitizer. Washing your hands should take 40 to 60 seconds, or how long it takes to sing the "Happy Birthday" song twice.

Here are the World Health Organization's seven steps to handwashing:

Step 1. Wet your hands and apply enough liquid soap to create a good lather.

Step 2. Rub your palms together.

Step 3. Rub the back of your hands.

Step 4. Interlink your fingers.

Step 5. Cup your fingers.

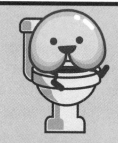

BUTTY'S SIDENOTE

Studies have shown that toilet water droplets, also known as toilet plume, can reach a distance of 6 feet when flushing!

Step 6. Clean your thumbs.

Step 7. Rub your palms with your fingers.

For hand sanitizer, the FDA gives you five important points to remember.

1. Rub a generous amount of sanitizer all over of your hands.

2. Make sure to get it between your fingers.

3. Make sure to rub the back of your hands.

4. Let the hand sanitizer dry naturally. There's no need to wipe or rinse it off.

5. Don't use sanitizer if your hands are noticeably dirty or greasy; wash with soap and water.

Your entire poop session should take no longer than 10 minutes.

Congratulations! You've completed a successful poop session. It should always be pain free and wonderfully relaxing. Oh, what a relief it is!

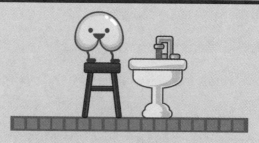

BUTTY'S ADDITIONAL TIPS FOR CLEANLINESS

When in public, try to avoid touching unnecessary surfaces. Avoid touching your face, which includes:

- Rubbing your eyes
- Picking your nose
- Touching your mouth

All these locations are vulnerable for germ transmission. Also remember these tips:

- Don't bite your nails.
- Regularly clip your nails.
- Avoid fake nails and fingernail polish, which can often breed bacteria.
- Protect any exposed cuts on your hands.

By following these hygiene tips, you are contributing directly to a cleaner environment for yourself and those around you.

REVIEW YOUR SUPPLEMENTS FOR ADVERSE GUT EFFECTS

As I mentioned in Chapter 3, several supplements may provide constipation relief. However, even natural supplements can cause unwanted side effects. Many of us take daily supplements in the form of multivitamins, multiminerals, omega-3 oils, soluble fiber, and herbs for a variety of other health benefits. The majority of these supplements, when taken in the recommended dosage, can be beneficial to your overall health. Nutritional supplements make up a multibillion-dollar industry that is not regulated by the FDA, so their efficacy is not always known. For that reason, it is important for you to know their potential benefits as well as the risks. In specific formulations, some supplements may cause gut problems, whereas those in a different formulation may be completely safe for you.

Here are a few examples of vitamins, minerals, and herbs that can cause gastric disturbances:

- High doses of vitamin D, iron, and calcium supplements can cause constipation.
- Conversely, high doses of vitamin C, certain forms of magnesium, and some herbal weight-loss supplements with senna, cascara, and rhubarb root can cause diarrhea.

It's always best to follow the dosing instructions on the labels because you'll be less likely to have unwanted gastric side effects. If you take the recommended dosages and still have gut issues, then discontinue the use of the suspected culprits. If your poop issues are serious, consult a trusted medical professional to help you resolve them.

REVIEW YOUR MEDICATIONS FOR UNWANTED SIDE EFFECTS

Take an inventory of all the medications you are currently using. You might be surprised at how many of them can affect your precious plumbing network, as well as the quality of your poops. Be proactive and check the labels for possible side effects, and do your own research if you suspect your poop problems may be related to a medication you take. It is common knowledge that opiates, antacids with calcium, the overuse of laxatives, and some antidepressants like Zoloft can cause constipation. On the loose end of the poop scale, certain antibiotics, some antacids, and proton-pump inhibitors such as omeprazole can cause diarrhea. It's also good to be aware that if you are treated with chemotherapeutic agents, depending on the type, you can get either diarrhea or constipation. Consult with your medical professional if you suspect that your difficulties pooping may be directly related to the effects of one or more of your medications. Oftentimes, another medication can be substituted for the offending one and still be effective for you without the gut-disturbing side effects.

I'll bet you didn't know there were so many simple tools to help you poop better! All it takes is for you to start using them, little by little, until they become part of your everyday routine. Then, you won't know how you lived without them. Like I said before, knowledge is power, and in this case, knowledge is poop power in action!

CHAPTER 6

LIFESTYLE CHOICES FOR THE JOY OF POOPING

"It is health that is real wealth and not pieces of gold and silver."
—Mahatma Gandhi, 20th-century leader of Indian nationalism

ELLA'S STORY: FINDING OUT THE TRUTH

Ella arrives at the Regional Medical Center a few minutes early and finds her way to the imaging clinic. After a short wait, she is greeted by Nurse Valdez, who escorts her to a spacious room with a large scanning machine. She explains to Ella that the machine is a specialized X-ray imaging device that will be used to scan her pelvic floor to detect or rule out any anomalies. Nurse Valdez tells her that this procedure, involving a continual series of X-rays, is called an X-ray defecography. Ella is vaguely familiar with what's to happen next because she received an email from Dr. Sloan's office instructing her not to urinate one hour before the appointment and to try to poop the night before to empty her rectum. She was able to do this, despite being perplexed at the odd, skinny hook-shaped turds that eventually came out.

Ella listens intently as Nurse Valdez further explains that she will be sitting down over a type of toilet, her bare butt and privates covered with a sheet, while the X-ray scanner captures several images. Ella's rectum will be filled with a special contrast barium paste that will enhance dynamic images of her pelvic floor while at rest, when she squeezes and strains, and when she poops the paste out, so that an accurate picture of her rectal and anal structures and functions can be documented in real time.

Once informed of the entire process, Ella, though nervous, feels ready to proceed with the test. She is hopeful that the X-ray scans will help Dr. Sloan figure out why she is still constipated and why she often feels there is more poop in her rectum that won't come out. The imaging procedure is successful and takes 30 minutes from start to finish. Nurse Valdez praises Ella for doing a great job. She feels relieved after excreting the paste and letting go of the tension that had built up in anticipation of the imaging process.

The next day, Ella arrives fifteen minutes early for her appointment with Dr. Sloan. She quickly fills out the history and HIPAA forms and gives them to the receptionist. Ella nervously flips through a golf magazine as she waits to be called back. After thirty minutes, a nurse calls her back, checks her vitals, escorts her to a clinic room, and asks her to put on a paper gown and remove her underwear.

After another 10 minutes, Dr. Sloan, a tall, slender man in a white lab coat with gray hair and a full beard, comes in and greets Ella in a friendly manner. He asks her to tell him what's going on with her gut as he looks over her history form. Once he's finished with the questions, he informs her that his next step is to perform a digital exam of her anus and rectum. He asks Ella to bend over the examining table with her butt facing him, then he gloves up, lubricates his left forefinger, and carefully inserts it into her anus and rectum. He probes around for physical abnormalities and is finished in a couple of minutes. Afterward, he tells Ella that he detects something odd with the structure of her rectum, and he wants to order some other tests before giving her a definitive diagnosis.

The next procedure for Ella is an anorectal manometry performed by a nurse practitioner named Gloria. Gloria preps Ella with lubricant, inserts a narrow, flexible tube in her anus and rectum, and then inflates a small balloon on the end of the tube. The device is then pulled back through the anal sphincter to allow a measurement to be taken of the way her muscles coordinate to move her bowels. The results are recorded on a computer screen. Gloria concurrently performs an electromyography (EMG) recruitment test during the manometry procedure to measure the electrical activity of the pelvic floor muscles. After she completes the procedures, Gloria informs Ella that as soon as Dr. Sloan has had a chance to look at the images and test results, he will discuss the findings with her. She is then directed back to the clinic room, where Dr. Sloan first examined her.

After forty minutes of waiting, Ella hears Dr. Sloan lightly knock on the door before he enters the clinic room. As expected, she is anxious to hear what he has to say. He tells her that he has just received the X-ray defecography results, along with the manometry and EMG findings, and that the test results confirmed his suspicion from the digital exam. As he shows her the dynamic X-ray imaging, he explains that she has a mild rectocele, or prolapse of her rectum into the vaginal wall, and tells her this is fairly common in females. "In plain English, this means that, due to the straining you did trying to poop, you stretched your rectum and created a small internal pouch that, when filled with poop, pushes on the back wall of your vagina. Some of your poop gets trapped in that little pouch, which is why you have abdominal pain and often feel like you have to go, but can't. This is also why your stools are often skinny with a hook shape on one end."

Ella nods her head as things finally start to make sense to her. After a brief pause, she asks Dr. Sloan if she will need surgery to correct the problem. He replies that because the recto-cele is mild, he is confident that with biofeedback therapy in his clinic, combined with dietary and lifestyle changes, she can learn how to control her pelvic muscles so she can poop properly and get her life back on track without the need for surgery. He explains that it will take a strong desire and a great deal of self-discipline on her part to make the changes needed to succeed and avoid surgery down the road.

EXAMPLES OF NORMAL PELVIC FLOOR AND RECTOCELE (PELVIC ORGAN PROLAPSE)

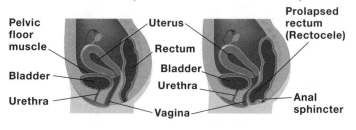

NORMAL ANATOMY   RECTOCELE

Before Dr. Sloan moves on to his next patient, he coun-sels Ella to start eating a high-fiber diet and drinking plenty of water each day. He instructs her to stop taking laxatives, start taking two psyllium fiber capsules, and take one or two

probiotic tablets with each meal. He recommends that she
work out regularly or at least get some form of daily exercise
for twenty minutes each day and stop pushing and straining
when she poops. Before leaving the clinic, Ella schedules six
more appointments, one per week for the next six weeks, for
biofeedback therapy sessions.

GOOD DIET—NO EXERCISE

We spent a lot of time looking at the good, the bad, and
the ugly of food and drink consumption in the last chapter.
You can have the healthiest, hydrated, fiber-filled, lean protein, carbohydrate-balanced diet in the world and still have
problems pooping *if* you are a person who doesn't get up and
move on a daily basis!

Exercise is a critical component of maintaining a healthy gut.
Daily mild to moderate exercise reduces the time it takes for
food to move through your large intestine (colon). Exercise
limits the quantity of water absorbed from your stools, which
allows them to pass more quickly and easily without becoming
hard and dry. Aerobic exercises accelerate your heart rate
and breathing, which helps stimulate the natural contractions
(peristalsis) of your intestinal muscles, and allows stools to
move through your gut more speedily and efficiently. Let's not
forget the effects of simple gravity with movement. If we are

sitting and not moving much all day, the effects of gravity and movement to help the waste pass through your gut are limited.

It seems that our society has become more sedentary than ever before, with a plethora of visual and auditory information coming to us from all sides via our cell phones, tablets, laptops, PCs, HD TVs, and gaming arrays. Don't get me wrong, the use of digital technology with lightning-fast speeds has given us more safety features in our vehicles and homes, more precise medical equipment to fight disease, and faster and easier communication with our loved ones and friends from all around the world. But it can hamper our motivation to get up and move if we can binge-watch a new series, get the news, watch sports, keep up with friends on social media, or play any number of games practically anywhere we are.

Even though we are supposedly the most intelligent animals on the planet, we seem to forget that we have a body with arms, legs, hands, feet, hundreds of muscles and bones, thousands of nerve fibers, a huge network of arteries and veins, trillions of cells and microbes, an exquisite plumbing system for digestion and excretion, five senses, and a brain that all require oxygen-rich blood, nutrient-rich food, hydration for energy, and *movement* to keep us strong and healthy.

THE POWER OF **Pooping**

FOUR KEY LIFESTYLE CHOICES FOR BETTER POOPING

Your lifestyle is how you choose to live your life—what you eat and drink, what activities you fill your days with, what you believe or don't believe, what you like and don't like, how you make your living, and how you maintain relationships with your family, loved ones, friends, teachers, coworkers, and pets.

Since I'm focusing on pooping, let's take a look at four simple lifestyle choices/changes, along with your diet, that can help you realize the power of pooping in your life.

STRESS MANAGEMENT

Stress management can help to calm your body, mind, and emotions and help you rebalance. Keep in mind there are many different techniques for stress management. A technique I personally use is a modified form of Nadi Shodhana Pranayama, also called alternate nostril breathing. Check out how to do this online at banyanbotanticals.com.

I also find being in the present moment helps reduce stress. Worrying and reflecting too much is never helpful for calming the mind.

To help ease worrying, start journaling your thoughts, emotions, present and future goals, and gratitude for all the good things in your life.

BUTTY'S BONUS TIPS\

If you are sixty or older, there are many resources on the best type of exercises for you, such as "5-Exercises Seniors Should Do Every Day" on YouTube or "7 Best Exercises for Seniors" from seniorlifestyle.com. There are also many online exercise resources for those who have bad knees, bad backs, arthritis, or other issues.

Others use meditation as a form of stress relief. This could include the following:

- Calming music
- Meditation through focused breathing
- Meditation via exercise
- Visualization exercises (imagining you're in a safe, inviting place)

THE POWER OF **Pooping**

SLEEP

Sleep plays an important role in both your physical and mental health. It also has a major effect on your poop health! Here are some tips to ensure quality sleep:

- Create a regular sleep schedule. This will help you go to bed at the same time every night and wake up at the same time every morning. Keep the same sleep schedule—even on weekends!

- Have regularly scheduled meals.

  - Make every effort to eat your meals at the same time each day.

  - Feel free to modify your foods to best fit your needs. For instance, if you are lactose intolerant, use lactose-free dairy products. If you have a food allergy, avoid that food and substitute something else for it.

  - Avoid eating heavy meals right before bed, but don't go to sleep hungry either. I find it helpful to have a glass of warm milk and/or a banana an hour before bed to help me sleep through the night.

  - Be mindful to avoid caffeine, sugar, and heavy carbs before bed.

- Limit artificial lights at least one hour before bedtime. This includes cell phones, TVs, and other screens.

- Try to sleep an average of eight to nine hours per night.

STRETCH AND EXERCISE

You should exercise for at least twenty minutes per day. Remember to stretch before and after you exercise!

Two great forms of exercise are:

Aerobic (cardio): hiking, biking, swimming

Anaerobic: involves more intense bursts of physical activity, like weight lifting or high-intensity interval training

You don't have to be a professional athlete, just get moving! This could include:

- Cleaning your home
- Walking in the park
- Taking your dog for a walk around the neighborhood
- Taking the stairs instead of the elevator
- If you sit for long periods of time, taking stretch breaks 5 to 10 minutes every hour
- Doing hamstring stretches and touching your toes

Other great forms of exercise with stretching include:

- Yoga
- Pilates
- Tai chi

146   THE POWER OF *Pooping*

LIMIT SUBSTANCE USE

Avoid or limit your intake of recreational drugs. If you decide to partake, be prepared to deal with the side effects. Substances that can affect your delicate plumbing system include:

Nicotine tobacco products. They are a major factor of risk for peptic ulcers, Crohn's disease, damage to the gut lining, and immune responses of the gut, according to the National Center for Biotechnology Information at the NIH.

Vaping. UC San Diego's Department of Cellular and Molecular Medicine found that vaping can break down the gut lining, triggering inflammation and leading to inflammatory bowel disease.[23]

Cannabis. Cannabis in certain forms and doses can have health benefits, but long-term use and/or high doses can cause abdominal pain, vomiting, and nausea.

CBD products. In strong dosages, these can cause GI disturbances, including diarrhea and appetite loss.

Alcohol. In moderate to large quantities, alcohol can attack the lining of the stomach and esophagus and cause ulcers,

---

23 Jeanna Vasquez, "Study: E-Cigarettes Trigger Inflammation in the Gut," UC San Diego News Center, January 7, 2021, https://ucsdnews.ucsd.edu/archives/date/070121.

nausea, and intestinal damage. It has also been a causative link to colon cancer.

Caffeine. Caffeine can cause increased gut motility that can lead to diarrhea and anxiety, which can make gut conditions like inflammatory bowel disease (IBD), or disorders encompassing chronic inflammation of your digestive tract, and IBS worse.

These products also have many other side effects that can affect your energy levels, mood stability, mental clarity, sleep quality, and more.

For example, caffeine and nicotine are stimulants, which can initially provide you with energy. But an unwanted side effect is that when a stimulant wears off, you need to have more. These stimulants can also increase your stress levels.

Although alcohol can initially produce a stimulant effect, it is a depressant. It can lower your normal energy level and exacerbate your daily stressors, particularly if it is used to cope with stress, which can lead to heavier drinking and alcoholism. This in turn leads to changes in brain chemistry, loss of self-care, and reduced social and cognitive awareness.

Side effects can include a disruption of the following:

- Mood
- Quality of sleep

- Appetite, impacting nutrition

- Physical energy

- Mental clarity

Marijuana can also have unwanted side effects, such as:

- Short-term memory loss

- Nausea

- Dehydration

- Reduced sleep quality

- Anxiety and paranoia

Do your homework before ingesting any of the above products, especially in high doses. And remember, health is your real wealth!

CREATE YOUR OWN POOP SCHEDULE

Do you always have to poop at the worst possible times of the day? I'll bet you didn't know that you can actually train your digestive system to poop at specific times of the day. A poop schedule is a predictable time in the day when you can have regular bowel movements.

You can schedule your poops:

- In the morning before showering

- In the evenings before bedtime

- Or whenever it's most convenient for you

The first step in creating a poop schedule is to assess your daily routine. First ask yourself, "What is my current daily poop schedule?" Then follow up with these questions:

- When do I wake up?

- When do I bathe or shower?

- When do I eat, drink, and go to sleep?

- And most importantly, when do I usually poop?

Now that you have the basic idea of your daily schedule, you can narrow down when you want to poop. A lot of my patients find it most convenient to poop in the morning before work, while some prefer the afternoon and others at night before bed. But ultimately, you need to pick a time when you have the ability to be in a relaxed state of mind, with some minutes to spare.

What time of day is the most convenient for you? Once you answer that question, you can begin setting your new poop schedule with the following habits.

Eat at a scheduled time every day, which includes breakfast, lunch, and dinner. Our body thrives on routines. By eating at scheduled times each day, your gut will establish a regular bowel pattern.

Sleep at a scheduled time. Be sure to sleep every night and wake up every morning at similar times. This allows your body to establish a pattern for hunger, sleep, energy level, and most importantly, pooping!

Move around before pooping. Be active around the house or workplace, or engage in light to moderate exercise. By moving your body around, you stimulate peristalsis, which shifts your food down the digestive tract. Being active, rather than sedentary, allows gravity to stimulate your gut.

Give yourself a window of time to relax and poop in peace. This should be around fifteen to thirty minutes before pooping. Make sure you are calm and in the right mindset to poop. Being in a stressful environment *never* helps when you're trying to relax and poop. When pooping, you should be on the toilet for a *maximum of 10 minutes without straining or pushing.*

All of these changes combined will allow you to have the *perfect* poop schedule. Don't worry if this doesn't work on the first day! Remember, *consistency* is key. If you have normal gut health, you should be able to establish this within two to seven days. If you are still having problems, consult with your GI or colorectal physician.

SAMPLE POOP SCHEDULE
MORNING POOPER

Time	Action
7:00 a.m.	Wake up
7:00–7:30 a.m.	Brief stretches, then 20 minutes of aerobic/anaerobic exercise Drink at least 8 ounces of water
7:30 a.m.	Breakfast
8:00 a.m.	Poop
8:15 a.m.	Shower and get ready for the day
12:00 p.m.	Lunch
6:00 p.m.	Dinner
8:00 p.m.	Yoga exercises and stretching
9:00 p.m.	Meditate
10:00 p.m.	Sleep

EVENING POOPER

Time	Action
8:00 a.m.	Wake up
8:00–8:15 a.m.	Brief stretches Drink at least 8 ounces of water
8:30 a.m.	Breakfast
12:00 p.m.	Lunch
6:00 p.m.	Dinner
8:00 p.m.	Yoga exercises and stretching, or any form of exercise you like
8:30 p.m.	Poop
8:45 p.m.	Shower and wind down
11:00 p.m.	Sleep

BLANK SCHEDULE

Fill in your own poop schedule here:

Time	Action

MOTIVATION IS YOUR KEY TO SUCCESS

Lack of motivation for making wholesale lifestyle changes is probably the biggest obstacle I encounter from my patients, even if they want to escape the vicious cycle of constipation. I (and other medical professionals) can perform all the special tests needed to help them understand their specific problems and counsel them till I'm blue in the face, but if they aren't motivated to take that first step to help themselves, then the odds are that their issues with constipation will continue to haunt them for a very long time. Perhaps it's the fear of getting out of their comfort zone, despite the misery they are in. Maybe they're lazy, in a rut, or simply lack the self-discipline to improve their condition. These patients sadden me because they are missing out on the joy of pooping and an overall better quality of life.

On the flip side, I am inspired and heartened by my patients who are motivated to do whatever it takes to improve their condition. I call them my "rock stars" because no matter what obstacles they face, they keep a positive attitude, take the necessary steps to change their lifestyle, and focus on achieving the goal of better poop health. There is nothing more gratifying to me than hearing returning patients' success stories! I love to see the joy on their faces when they realize that, because of their desire and self-discipline (and a little help from me), everything came out beautifully in the end!

CHAPTER 7

FEEL THE POWER OF POOPING!

"All good poops which exist are the fruits of originality."
—John Stuart Mill, 19th-century British philosopher

ELLA'S STORY: GETTING HER LIFE BACK

Ella is relieved to finally know why she's had so much trouble pooping and that, if she follows Dr. Sloan's directives, she won't need surgery. Rather than let this new-found knowledge and understanding of her condition drag her down, Ella feels an energy rising from somewhere deep within her consciousness. It's a power she has never felt before, a power that vibrates through her entire being, enveloping her in a warm blanket of love. It wordlessly tells her that she is loved, she matters, and her very existence depends on the choices she makes moving forward.

This power, with its unspoken words, jolts Ella into realizing how much she has ignored her body's cries for help, how she has put her health last on her list of priorities, and how, instead of loving herself, she has abused the precious gift of life with its rich opportunities for growth on so many levels. This revelation becomes the catalyst that spurs Ella to start loving and valuing her body, mind, emotions, and spirit. Ella will start doing everything she can to create a new life, vibrant with health and happiness!

The first person Ella calls after seeing Dr. Sloan is her mother. Rather than blubbering like a lost child as she did a few weeks back, she calmly tells her mom about all the tests performed on her and the doctor's finding of a mild rectocele. She also tells Diana how motivated she is to get healthy again and to get her life back. Diana is relieved to know the diagnosis and that surgery isn't required. She senses that something has changed in her daughter. Instead of trepidation, Diana feels strength and confidence exuding from Ella's tone of voice. After chatting a while longer, mother and daughter come to the conclusion that Ella should try to take six to eight weeks off from her job so she can focus all of her time and energy on getting and staying healthy.

Ella returns to work the following day and is able to have a sit-down with her boss. Putting all embarrassment aside, she opens up about her medical condition and the agony she has endured over the past month. She tells him how important she feels it is to use her accumulated four weeks of sick leave, two weeks of vacation time, and two weeks of leave without pay to attend the biofeedback therapy sessions and gradually make changes to her diet and lifestyle so she can learn to manage her condition. She also asks him not to tell anyone else in the office about her health issue, which he readily agrees to. After hearing her heartfelt story, surprisingly, Ella's boss approves her request but asks her to compromise at seven weeks of time off with the option of a one-week extension if she needs more time to take care of her problem. Even though she knows there's a long way to go to get her health and life back on track, Ella is elated after the heart-to-heart and subsequent leave approval from her boss.

Now it's time to get to work. With the goal of preserving the integrity of her rectum sans surgery and relearning how to poop without straining, Ella is laser-focused on learning everything she can about her condition and how to manage it. She searches the internet to gather as much information as she possibly can and discovers an online support group for women with rectoceles. Ella reads several stories on this particular website from women who opted for surgical repair of their rectoceles as well as from those who did the work to learn how to manage them.

The following Monday is Ella's first session with an advanced nurse whose specialty is biofeedback therapy. Nurse Lee warmly welcomes Ella to her clinic, asks a few questions about her condition for better clarity, then explains what bio-feedback of the pelvic floor muscles entails. She tells Ella how it will help her, over time, learn when and how to contract and relax the muscles of her rectum and anus so she should never again have to resort to pushing and straining to poop. She also explains that, even with the small internal pouch from the rectocele, if Ella makes the necessary changes to her diet and lifestyle, she will be free of constipation and should be able to relax and poop with relative ease.

After Nurse Lee finishes the biofeedback session, she explains the benefits of using electrical stimulation, another form of therapy, which she plans to add to the sessions. She tells Ella that she will teach her how to use it in the clinic. Later on, Ella will have the option of purchasing her own device for home use to help strengthen as well as relax her anal/rectal muscles. Ella feels so blessed to have such a caring mentor that she affectionately begins calling Nurse Lee her "Poop Doula," which delights everyone in the clinic. In addition to facilitating the biofeedback and electrical stimulation therapy, Nurse Lee continually counsels Ella about many simple tools she can use to improve her pooping experience.

Over the next six weeks, in addition to her once-a-week bio-feedback sessions, Ella makes wholesale changes to her daily routine. She goes to bed each night and gets up in the morning at the same times. She stretches and works out at the gym every day, combining both aerobic and anaerobic exercises. Ella surprises herself by giving up all caffeinated drinks after one week of withdrawal headaches and begins hydrating her body with six to eight glasses of water a day. Along with cutting out caffeine, she quits drinking alcoholic beverages, except for an occasional glass of red wine with dinner.

One of the biggest changes, besides nixing the caffeine, is to Ella's diet. She finds a website that lays out a seven-day meal plan that closely matches Dr. Sloan's recommendations of a high-fiber diet with vegetables, fruits, whole grains, fish rich in omega-3 oils, shellfish, and a small amount of lean meat once or twice a week. She takes two psyllium capsules and one probiotic tablet with billions of good guy bacteria in them with each meal.

Ella expects to see results, but they come sooner than she thought. After only three weeks of biofeedback therapy, changing her diet, getting plenty of sleep, and exercising, she realizes that she is pooping like she's never pooped before! She poops at least once, usually twice, and occasionally three times a day! Now, as soon as she feels the urge, she sits on the pot, blows lightly three times on a tissue, and with grace and ease, the rich, full-bodied, banana-shaped turds literally slide out of her anus within five to eight minutes of sitting down. She is now able to empty her rectum without the lingering sensation of more poop inside that won't come out. Ella quickly begins to feel such an amazing sense of relief every time she poops that she actually starts looking forward to her time on the pot each day! (Her previous practice of pushing and straining soon becomes a distant memory.)

In addition to the biofeedback therapy and diet and lifestyle changes, Ella starts keeping a journal. At the end of every day, about ten to fifteen minutes before bedtime, she closes her eyes, contemplates on her daily interactions and her gratitude for the gifts as well as the tests in her life, then records these along with her thoughts, hopes, and dreams for the future as a way to stay in a relaxed, positive state of mind. After four weeks of journaling before bed each night, she becomes aware that she is having some awesome dreams, so she knows she's entering the deep sleep cycle called rapid eye movement (REM). She knows from her online research that the REM cycle of sleep is when she is getting the best quality rest for optimal rejuvenation of the cells and organs of her body.

The six weeks of biofeedback therapy, four of which include electrical stimulation, go by quickly. Soon after the fourth ses-

sion, Ella purchases an electrical stim device for home and starts using it religiously once a day. At the last session, Nurse Lee informs Ella that she has reached the pinnacle of rock star success! Indeed, the progress she's made in such a short time is remarkable. Before Ella leaves the clinic on that final day, Nurse Lee tells her she'll be right back. She returns with a "diploma" in an official-looking font that she printed out with the date, Ella's name, and a statement that says Ella has met all the requirements for an advanced degree in "Poopatology." When she hands it to Ella, they both break out in laughter and give each other a big hug. Ella thanks Nurse Lee for her kindness and for everything she has taught her during those six weeks, then leaves the clinic to go home.

Ella's seven weeks away from work give her a new perspective on herself and her place in the world. With plenty of time to think and reflect upon her career path, she asks herself "Do I really want to continue working in a stress-filled, pressure-cooker environment, where I might start slipping and return to the old pattern of neglecting my health?" Her answer was a resounding no!

After witnessing the compassion and caring nature of the health-care professionals who helped her get through her crisis, Ella decides she wants to pursue a more meaningful career, where she can give back to others and to the planet. In college, she graduated with a double major in computer science and ecology. She took the first job she was offered because of the high-paying salary and the scarcity of work related to ecology. From a young age, Ella has always had a profound respect for the environment, as well as concern about the effects of global warming.

Upon gaining this newfound love and respect for her body, Ella decides she's going to give notice at work that she will be leaving in a few weeks to pursue a new career. With more and more companies being formed to find creative solutions to the consequences of global warming and its effects on people around the globe, Ella is more excited than ever to enter a new chapter of her life. In hindsight, she is grateful for the health crisis she eventually faced and overcame with the help of caring medical professionals, for it woke her up to a new horizon of greater possibilities for a brighter future. And most of all, it taught her how the precious gift of vibrant health should never be taken for granted.

In the end, Ella fully realizes the power of pooping in her life. Over time, it leads her to a richer future imbued with health and happiness, treasures far greater than gold and silver.

CLOSING THOUGHTS

Ella's story is inspiring and parallels that of so many of my patients who are willing to do the work changes to free their lives from the grips of debilitating gut problems and avoid going under the knife. Of course, not all of their stories are like Ella's. I know that not all of my patients have the luxury of taking long periods of time off from work or changing careers, depending on their age and health status, but it's important to know that help is available.

Many of the patients I see have conditions that have deteriorated to the point that, often, and through no fault of their own, surgery is necessary and lifesaving. My hat goes off to the dedicated GIs, colorectal physicians, surgeons, and support staff who go the extra mile every day to help patients make the hard decisions that give them a chance to live the best lives they can.

I am so blessed to be in a position to help and hopefully inspire people to experience the positive benefits of the power of pooping. I used to be embarrassed to tell new acquaintances what I do for a living because of the reactions they might have. But when I reflect upon all the special people I have met and helped throughout my long career, I feel a profound sense of gratitude and pride for the opportunity and honor to have served them.

Now, for those of you who suffer from constipation and still feel as if you need more help, the next section of the book gives you some practical meal plans. These will make it easier to start working on the all-important changes needed to feel the awesome power of pooping in your own life. Before you start making big changes to your diet and lifestyle, you need to prepare yourself psychologically for a whole new way of living and work into it slowly. This requires you to be motivated enough to commit to creating a healthier poop life.

For more information on all aspects of poop health, check out the *Butt Talks* team's website at ButtTalksTV.com.

Have a great poop day!

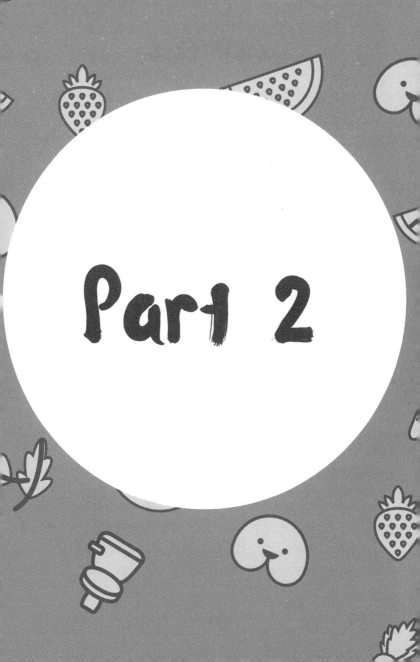

Part 2

CHAPTER 8

PREPARATIONS FOR EATING HEALTHY

"Let food be thy medicine and medicine be thy food."
—Hippocrates, ancient Greek physician regarded as the father of medicine

It is my hope that you enjoyed and learned something from Ella's story as well as from the information passed along to you in the first section of this book. I hope it gave you some insight into how your digestive system works, why it doesn't work so well at times, and how you can live a healthier, happier life through the power of pooping.

In this section of the book, I will share some practical tips for eating healthy on a budget, as well as some sample meal plans so you can get your daily fiber, protein, and essential nutrients to better realize the power of pooping.

PRACTICAL TIPS FOR EATING ON A BUDGET

Every time you think of eating healthy, you may say to yourself, how is that possible? It is easier than you think. It doesn't mean that you need to spend a ton of money either. It may require you to make some of your meals at home, but in the long run, it is cheaper and more nutritious, and you can be the boss of your stomach!

Trust me. Your bowels will love you and you them!

The following sections break out some tips, tricks, and best practices to have the foods you need in a well-organized kitchen.

Basics. A well-stocked pantry includes grains, beans, and whole grain bread. Also, keep basic items in your fridge, like the milk of your choice, whether cow, goat, soy, almond, or oat; eggs; unsweetened yogurt made from the milk of your choice; lean meats; fruits; veggies; and salsa. Finally, stock up on the likes of organic miso paste, pesto sauce, and tomato paste to add flavor to your dishes.

Organization and roommates. Do you share an apartment or house with roommates? If so, you will need adequate space for your food so no one will eat it before you get to it. Establish some rules with your roommates so they are respectful of your food. You can easily post a list of your items in a common area, or, better yet, establish a designated space for each roomie to keep their own food.

You may want to label your refrigerated items by marking your name on a piece of painter's or masking tape or putting a note on the outside of the fridge to identify your items. This can help avoid the possibility of territorial disputes!

Storage. Proper storage is important to keep all foods fresh and easy to identify. Separate bins with sealed lids are helpful to store dried bulk items, such as pinto, navy, and other beans; whole grains like oatmeal, quinoa, whole grain pasta, and rice; and sweeteners like honey, stevia, or cane sugars. Buying nonperishable dried foods in bulk can save you money in the long run. Many food co-ops and some grocery stores provide bulk foods, herbs, and spices in large bins so you can purchase as much or as little as you wish.

Keep perishable but longer-lasting vegetables such as potatoes, onions, garlic, and yams in other containers, but keep special considerations for these items in mind. For instance, if you don't store your potatoes correctly, they can turn soft and green, grow sprouts, mold or get rotten, and turn juicy and smelly! This means it is time to toss them out or put them in the ground to grow a new crop of potatoes! The goal is to eat the slightly sprouted tubers first and keep them stored properly in an open bowl or a well-ventilated paper or cloth bag. Try to eat starchy foods (carbs) in moderation, as the starch turns into sugar, which can contribute to the development of body fat.

If potatoes develop a green color on the skin then there's most likely a high level of glycoalkaloids, which can make them taste bitter and cause a burning irritation in the back of your mouth and side of your tongue. Besides that, glycoalkaloids can affect the nervous system and cause major GI discomfort. When your potatoes turn green and develop sprouts, it's time to toss them out and perhaps limit how many you buy in the future.

Make sure to store eggs properly by leaving them in the store-bought container and putting them on the middle shelf of your fridge, NOT in the plastic holder of your fridge door. For the sake of your safety, be sure to read and observe the expiration date on the carton. The most commonly associated germ that leads to food poisoning from eggs is salmonella. This can come from fecal matter on the eggshells and even from hens with salmonella-infected ovaries. Strict cleaning and inspection of eggs as well as regular tests on the hens for salmonella has kept possible outbreaks on an industry level at bay, although they can still occur. Keep your eggs in the refrigerator at 40 degrees or lower. Don't use eggs that are cracked, damaged, or semi-cooked. If you purchase or make egg-based foods, they must be refrigerated within two hours of preparation. For recipes like pasta carbonara or original Caesar dressing that require partially uncooked eggs, use *only* pasteurized eggs.

Before I get into the storage of meats, poultry, and seafood, you should know that the storage times I've recommended are on the conservative side. You may be able to refrigerate and freeze some items a little longer than I suggested. If meat, poultry, or seafood is kept too long in the refrigerator or left out on the counter for over two hours uncooked, you can be subject to foodborne diseases that come in the form of bacteria, viruses, and parasites that can all seriously affect your gut and overall health. Make sure you are informed on the length of refrigeration for these types of foods. I highly recommend that you write the dates of expiration on everything you freeze. I remember visiting my elderly mother a few years ago over the holidays and finding items in her freezer chest labeled with the dates she froze them, but many of them were up to five years old! Needless to say, those items had to be quietly chucked when she was asleep.

When freezing beef, lamb, pork, poultry, or seafood, it is best to keep them in the original packaging, then put them in resealable freezer bags for optimal storage. If you plan to freeze items for several months, it's best to put frozen items in individual plastic freezer bags to help ward off freezer burn.

For comprehensive information on the proper storage of meats, fish, fruit, and vegetables go to foodsafety.gov.

CHEF BUTTY'S TIP ON TATERS AND TUBERS

Don't wash potatoes and tubers until you are ready to cook them or they will mold, and you will have wasted your money!

Best Practices: Carrots and other veggies need to be refrigerated or they will mold. Read the labels on the containers if you're unsure if refrigeration is needed.

Read and respect labels and expiration dates. Remember that canned goods also have a shelf life. If cans are dented, don't buy them! If the top of the can is bulging even slightly, there may be bacteria growing and pushing up the lid. If you don't see a bulge in a can until you get home, don't open it! Toss it out or return it to the store for a refund. The same goes for packaged foods, including refrigerated, vacuum-packed meats; if they feel puffy after having been in the refrigerator, they can be dangerous to open and eat. Many bacteria form a gas when they multiply, which leads to the puffy package.

If any food items, refrigerated or canned, have a foul odor, do not taste them! One slight brush with this can expose you to the dangerous bacterial pathogens it contains. Bacteria are often invisible to the naked eye, but are so concentrated and powerful they can knock you on your a** and make you very sick!

If you see mold on any food, toss it out! Mold looks like white or gray "cotton;" it is airborne and very potent. Isolating and containing mold before the spores go flying into your nose or mouth is critical! Wear gloves and always wash them and your hands of all these cooties after you handle them. This is the safest way to keep you from getting sick!

Meal planning and portions. When planning your meals to eat healthy for the entire day or week, you can save a lot of time by making a list and shopping for only the specific items you need. Feel free to be creative with your meal plans by adding herbs and spices and by cooking foods in different ways such as baking, steaming, or grilling veggies to serve alongside a protein, grains, and other foods that are healthy for you. The myplate.gov division of foods graphic can help you create delicious, balanced meals.

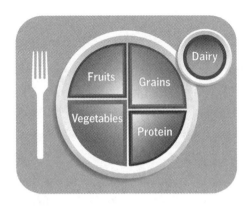

By following the myplate.gov template, you can figure out how much of each food you need for your meal plans. For guidance on the percentage of food types that help make up a healthy balanced meal, see page 117.

Cooking extra food will give you one or two meals for the next day or so. You can pack leftovers in a sealed container to carry to work or reheat later. This habit will save you time, extra decision-making, and money.

Figuring out protein portion sizes, like one thigh or drumstick, or a 4- to 5-ounce cut of lean meat or fish, will help you average out how many meals you need to carry you through the week. Family-size packages sold in grocery stores are usually cheaper than smaller packages. You can use the amount you need for a few days, then freeze the rest so you can have a different protein on other days. This, of course, depends on your taste and how much you want to vary your meals each week.

Buy for convenience. Ground meats are handy since they save on prep time required to trim or wash lean beef, turkey, or even the new ground meatless choices before cooking them. Just throw some into a pan and stir fry with your vegetables. Stretch out your portions with one-pot cooking that can cover most of the food categories. You can also pre-make some meatballs and cook them in a sauce to have leftovers for a few days, or freeze them for later.

Frozen fruits and veggies are convenient, and if they are flash-frozen, they maintain their nutritional value. It's great to have frozen organic strawberries on hand as they are so easy to put in the blender for a smoothie with blueberries or other fruits of your choice, protein powder, and whatever form of milk you prefer. Frozen veggies can be quickly stir-fried, steamed, or cooked in soups or casseroles.

Pickles, pineapple, applesauce, and other canned or bottled foods are handy and relatively inexpensive, but some contain added sugar, sodium, and preservatives. Read the list of ingredients to choose products with fewest additives.

You can elevate the taste of your dishes, such as rice and soup, by using vegetable or chicken broth as a base. You won't have to make the stock from scratch, just open a can or carton of beef or chicken broth (organic, low sodium, no sugar are best) and cook with some vegetables and—voilà—you can enjoy a lovely dish in minutes.

Nuts and dried fruits are great for enjoying on the go or as snacks at work. Buy them in bulk and measure out portions in small bags or containers to meet your dietary needs for the day. Some of these items are more expensive when pre-packaged.

Protein powders come in many different concentrated forms such as whey, soy, hemp, coconut, gluten-free grains, pea, and rice. Some of these protein powders are also fortified with digestive enzymes, probiotics, and additional fiber sources. Protein powders are considered a processed form of dietary supplement. It's important for you to know and understand that all protein powders are not created equally. The cheaper brands contain added sugars, artificial sweeteners, vegetable oils, and other additives. Besides that, the protein and extra vitamins and nutrients in any protein powder are not assimilated into your body as readily as protein from whole foods. It is always a good idea to do your homework and read the ingredients of any brand of protein powder to get the best quality before you make a purchase.

Herbs, spices, and condiments. A simple way to enhance the flavor of your foods and save money is to start your own herb garden. You can grow herbs on your kitchen windowsill or, if you live in a temperate climate like much of California, grow them in your yard or outside in a planter box. There's nothing quite as satisfying as reaping the benefits of freshly cut herbs at your fingertips!

You can also enjoy dried or frozen herbs and spices. They are easy to add and make your food taste so yummy! With the right choice of herbs and spices you won't want to go out to eat anymore, because most restaurants can't match the flavor of the herbs and spices in your home-cooked dishes. And you will definitely save money.

Be a little adventuresome with your foods. Keep some of the following seasonings on hand:

- Iodized salt, which is great for your thyroid, or kosher salt. These work well with most meats and dishes.

- Pepper, black or white, in a grinder or shaker.

- Spices like cinnamon, cumin, garlic powder, curry, garam masala, dill, red pepper flakes, paprika, thyme, rosemary, and many others make your foods much tastier.

Condiments such as reduced-fat mayonnaise, ground mustard, ketchup with minimal sugar, and butter or ghee are good to have in your refrigerator. For the cupboard, stock up on cold-pressed extra-virgin olive oil, some hot sauce like sriracha or Tabasco, soy sauce, Worcestershire sauce, tamari, and more to help add flavor and a little kick to your food.

If you are gluten or lactose intolerant, or if you have known food allergies, be sure you read the ingredients of all condiments to make sure they don't contain any of the offending culprits that may cause an unwanted reaction from you. Many soy sauces are derived from wheat products that contain gluten. Unless products containing dairy are in a lactose-free format, stay away from them if you are intolerant of lactose.

A friend's husband is allergic to the fairly common artificial taste enhancer, monosodium glutamate (MSG). It causes the airway to his lungs to constrict, making it harder for him to breathe. His wife always carries the antihistamine diphenhydramine (Benedryl) in her purse because, even after dining at very nice restaurants you wouldn't expect to use food additives, he has had unexpected reactions from MSG in the food. The diphenhydramine acts to open the airways and stifle the reaction. After a few of these incidents, he started carrying his own supply of this common over-the-counter medicine. If you are subject to severe allergic reactions called anaphylaxis, such as from MSG, peanuts, or eggs, you may need to carry an EpiPen to treat yourself immediately.

Basic kitchen utensils and accessories.

- Set of good kitchen knives

- Large cutting board

- Set of hot mitts to hold the handles on your pots

- Good set of nesting cooking pots for quick heat-ups

- Electric water kettle

- Basic set of dishes with bowls

- Basic set of forks, knives, and spoons

- Baking sheets

- Countertop electric convection oven

- Dishpan to soak your dishes or dirty utensils to start the cleaning process as you are cooking

- Supply of silicone gloves to handle raw meats and fish

- Paper towel holder

- Pair of sponges

* * *

Now that you have some ideas on how to eat healthier on a budget, along with several other food and kitchen tips, I'm going to give you some fairly simple, practical recipes and meal plans to help you with constipation, as well as with your overall health. Start using them today!

CHAPTER 9

RECIPES FOR CONSTIPATION RELIEF

"Whether the future looks scary or bright, plans are hopes made practical. They reassure people that there's a roadmap that will take them to a better place and they give people a reason to join in the effort to get there."

—Elizabeth Warren, from her book *Persist*

This section will give you five different breakfast, lunch, and dinner recipes. Having plenty of options to mix things up for you, your family, and friends is important to keep you from getting into meal ruts. It may also be important for some of you to create dishes that align with your cultural traditions as you cook and explore new healthier meal ideas using the tips from this book.

Each recipe I share will include the total fiber amount because fiber is the most poop-friendly ingredient! The amount of total fiber will be shown as a range since the use of optional ingredients will make the exact amount fluctuate.

For recipes that use protein powder, make sure to read the measurements located on the instruction label to determine the amount of protein in each serving. Some protein powders have added fiber from psyllium, flaxseed meal, and other sources. I personally use and recommend IsaLean meal-replacement protein powder by Isagenix.

As a reminder, see the Recommended Daily Fiber chart below for suggested fiber consumption by age and sex.[24]

RECOMMENDED DAILY FIBER

Age	Sex	Recommended Daily Fiber
1–3	Male and female	19 grams
4–8	Male and female	25 grams
9–13	Female	26 grams
9–13	Male	31 grams
14–19	Female	26 grams
14–19	Male	38 grams
20–50	Female	25 grams
20–50	Male	38 grams
Over 50	Female	25 grams
Over 50	Male	30 grams

24. Feliz J. Yangilar, "The Application of Dietary Fibre in Food Indsutry: Structural Features, Effects on Health and Definition, Obtaining and Analysis of Deitary Fibre," *Journal of Food and Nutrition Research* 1, no. 3 (2013): 13–23. https://doi.org/10.12691/jfnr-1-3-1.

The important thing to know about the ingredients in my recipes is that they are typically high in dietary fiber and geared to alleviate constipation, so you can experience the joy of pooping.

BREAKFAST

Fruit Smoothies

A morning smoothie is my breakfast staple. I make it large enough (20 to 32 ounces) to drink throughout the day. It's nutritious, easy to make, easy to bring with you in an insulated, portable bottle, and incredibly delicious, providing a balanced portion of fiber, protein, and amino acids. Many times at work or in social settings, the food available is low in fiber and causes constipation. Someone may order pizza for the office or your friends may ask you to go out to eat. You can save your smoothie to accompany lunch or dinner, or as a snack to ensure that you meet your daily fiber requirements by the end of the day.

Some people like to use juice or water as a base liquid, but I find that juice is too high in calories and sugar. Rather than grinding fruit fiber too finely, I recommend blending so that some texture is left to savor.

Starting your day off right with a tasty, nutritious smoothie, along with fiber and vitamin/mineral supplements, if used correctly, can support a better bowel movement pattern and address your constipation issues.

Prep time: 15 minutes | Cook time: 0 minutes | Makes: 2 (16-ounce) servings | Fiber Total: 12 to 20 grams

1 cup frozen strawberries or frozen fruit of choice, slightly thawed

½ cup fresh blueberries or fruit of choice, such as peaches, raspberries, or blackberries

¾ cup fresh greens, such as spinach (optional)

¼ cup protein powder

1 ripe banana, sliced

3 cups water or milk of your choice (2% milk can help you feel fuller longer)

½ cup plain unsweetened yogurt (optional)

1. Place the strawberries, or 1 cup of the frozen fruit of your choice, in the blender, then add ½ cup of blueberries or other fresh fruits. This is the best ratio of frozen to fresh fruits. Add ¾ cup of fresh greens, if using.

2. Add the protein powder to the mixture, then add the banana on top to weigh the powder down. This helps prevent the protein powder from clumping when you add liquid to the mixture. Both the banana and the protein powder will cut down some of the acidity of the other fruits so the smoothie isn't sour.

3. Pour in the milk or water, then blend.

4. Pour out the smoothies and enjoy! Serve yourself about 4 ounces with your morning breakfast. Bring it with you for the rest of the day to accompany your meals.

KEY FEATURES OF THIS DISH

- Liquid from fruits and the milk of your choice can keep you hydrated and support gut motility.

- Ideal pH levels from the balance of acidic fruits and base milk can lower gut irritation and keep you feeling full. It can help you avoid the urge to grab a bunch of snacks full of empty calories, and may help you cut down meal portions.

- Protein powder made from whey, vegetable sources, and/or collagen powder (beware vegans, collagen is made from animal by-products), as well as plain yogurt is a great source of an extra energy boost and essential amino acids that promote muscle and skin health and help you fight off certain free radicals (unstable atoms that can damage cells).

Nurse Wong's Morning Staple: Oatmeal

A breakfast standard, oatmeal is a hearty, low-fat meal that's full of antioxidants and protein to satisfy your hunger for three to four hours. This recipe uses rolled oats, though there are different categories of oats, which vary in texture and cut.

While categorized as a carbohydrate, oats are a very healthy whole grain packed with fiber, vitamins, and minerals that are essential for your nutritional health. Eating this simple breakfast ensures that your bowels will have the ingredients necessary to maintain good moisture.

Prep time: 15 minutes | Cook time: 2 minutes, 30 seconds | Makes: 2 (16-ounce) servings | Fiber Total: 15 to 18 grams

¼ cup dried rolled oats

1 tablespoon oat bran

1 tablespoon flaxseed meal

⅛ teaspoon ground cinnamon

1 teaspoon cane sugar, stevia, or agave syrup (optional)

1 cup boiling water

¾ cup fresh blueberries, divided

½ cup milk of choice

3 medium-sized chopped prunes (optional)

1. Mix the dried rolled oats, oat bran, flaxseed meal, cinnamon, and sweetener, if using, together in a large ceramic microwaveable bowl that can hold up to 2 cups of liquid.

2. Pour the boiling water in the bowl to quickly soften the mixture, then place the bowl into the microwave for 1 minute to add additional heat to the mixture.

3. Let stand for about 1 minute. The oats will soften and soak up all the water.

4. Add ¼ cup of blueberries and microwave again for another 30 seconds. Stir to mix and add the milk to cool.

5. Add the remaining ½ cup of fresh blueberries on top. You can also add a few prunes, which are a great choice for some extra sweetness and digestive benefits.

6. Enjoy the oatmeal while it's still warm!

KEY FEATURES OF THIS DISH

- **High-soluble fiber called beta-glucan gives oatmeal that creamy, gel-like texture and helps to form the ideal stool. Beta-glucan also helps with lowering cholesterol and blood sugar.**

- **Oatmeal increases the production of the satiety hormone to make you feel full longer, so it may help you eat fewer calories later in the day.**

Overnight Chia Seed Pudding

Chia seeds are a powerful source of nutritional goodness with a distinctive nutty flavor. They rehydrate quickly. One of the best ways to enjoy chia seeds is in overnight chia seed pudding—it is so easy to make, with no cooking involved.

The lighter your milk, the easier it will be for the chia seeds to soak it all up. Some light milk recommendations for this recipe are almond milk, soy milk, or 2 percent milk. For a heavier, thicker milk, you can mix it with some water to thin it down. (Avoid full-fat coconut milk, which is high in saturated fat.)

This tasty pudding will make you feel full and keep your tummy happy for quite a while.

Prep time: 5 minutes | Cook time: 5 minutes, plus overnight to set | Serves: 2 | Fiber Total: 17 to 19 grams

2 to 2½ tablespoons ground chia seeds

½ to 1 cup milk of choice

½ cup fresh fruit

1 ounce walnuts, granola, or nuts of choice (optional)

½ teaspoon honey, stevia, cane sugar, or agave nectar (optional)

1. Place the chia seeds in a 16-ounce jar or plastic container with a lid.

2. Add the milk. Depending on how creamy you want the pudding to be, you may choose to add more chia seeds to the mixture to get a thicker texture.

3. Mix the milk and chia seeds well with a spoon. Place the mixture in the refrigerator for 5 to 10 minutes, then stir again, picking up the bottom seeds with a spoon so they are equally hydrated and evenly distributed. This ensures a smooth and creamy texture the next day.

4. The next morning, add the fruits, walnuts or other toppings, if using, and sweetener, if you like. Enjoy!

CHEF BUTTY'S CHIA SEED TIP

Make sure you don't reverse steps 1 and 2. If you add the milk first and then the chia seeds, the chia seeds might end up floating on top of the milk and won't be able to absorb all the liquid well.

KEY FEATURES OF THIS DISH

- In addition to soluble fiber, chia seeds have the protein and gut-happy properties to create your delightful soft, creamy, full-figured future poops.

- Chia seeds soften and become gooey. This is a big bonus in helping your bowels stay together and stay soft.

- The prebiotic from the chia seeds help support good bacteria in the gut to help break down foods.

- Chia seeds have omega-3 fatty acids that help the body and bones absorb vitamins and nutrients. They are also helpful for heart health because they slow down the development of plaque in the arteries.

Overnight Oats

This meal, side dish, or dessert provides fiber to your daily diet—no cooking required! Take your overnight oats in a sealed container to work or school to support your bowel health and ensure that your stools will be creamy and luscious later. The grains in this recipe can help you feel fuller and reduce the need for snacks later in the day.

For the optional ingredients, you can be as creative as you wish by using what's in your kitchen. Just keep it healthy and limit the use of processed foods like cereal. The addition of flaxseed meal, chia seeds, or oat bran will increase your recipe to a much higher fiber content than just oatmeal alone.

This recipe can help you maintain bowel regularity and good nutrition with fiber, protein, and healthy fats.

Prep time: 10 minutes, plus overnight to refrigerate | Serves: 1 | Fiber Total: 27 to 30 grams

¼ cup rolled oats

½ to 1 cup no-sugar-added Greek yogurt, or yogurt of choice

1 tablespoon oat bran, flaxseed meal, or ground chia seeds (optional)

½ to 1 cup fresh or dried blueberries, raspberries, or fruit of choice

¼ to ½ cup milk of choice (optional)

1. Add the rolled oats to a medium container with a lid.

2. Layer the yogurt on top of the oats.

3. Add a thin layer of oat bran, flaxseed meal, or chia seeds, if using.

4. Add the fruit in equal portions so you are not eating more of one item than another. The key is to be balanced and have a little of everything that appeals to you. (You can also add the toppings from steps 3 and 4 after your oatmeal sets, prior to serving.)

5. Add milk, if using. This will make the mixture softer before putting in the fridge.

6. Refrigerate overnight.

KEY FEATURES OF THIS DISH

- The oats and yogurt supply fiber, enzymes, and live bacteria from probiotics (the good gut guys) to make your poop stay soft, rich, and creamy.

- Having a grain with fruits daily is helpful to keep your antioxidants at a gut-happy level.

Muesli and Overnight Muesli

Some people hate eating soft foods. They really like to chew something with many textures along with cold milk in the morning. Some people hate to even think about preparing anything in the morning except their coffee or tea so their eyelids can open a little wider. Then they think, "Should I eat something before I take off for work?" not knowing what kind of day lies ahead until they get there.

It is better that you eat a little something at home and take care of your business (poop) once the coffee or tea gets into your system. A bowl of healthy cereal—in this case, muesli—is best so you don't have to think about cooking anything for your breakfast. As another option, add a few tablespoons of Overnight Muesli to your fruit smoothies.

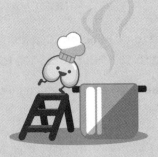

CHEF BUTTY'S BONUS TIPS

You can make a large amount of muesli to have on hand and store in a sealed jar or bin. Then you can use it to make the overnight version in this recipe.

Breakfast is different in many cultures; however, muesli can be a great cross-cultural breakfast food. It can help you poop at home before you start your day.

What is the difference between muesli and granola? **Muesli** contains raw grains, rolled oats, loose flakes, flaxseeds or flaxseed meal, wheat or oat bran, nuts, seeds, and dried fruits. The sugar in muesli is from the dried fruits. It is typically soaked overnight in milk or juice and served cold. **Granola** is made by mixing many of the same ingredients as muesli, but it contains oil and sweeteners that bind it together. Once mixed, it is baked to the crunchy consistency we are familiar with. Granola has a much higher sugar content, so muesli is the healthier choice of the two.

Dry Muesli

**Prep time: 20 to 30 minutes | Cook time: 0 minutes
| Serves: 10 to 15 | Fiber Total: 300 to 315 grams**

5 cups whole grain flakes (any combination of barley, quinoa, Kamut, rye, or spelt)

3¾ cups rolled oats

2 tablespoons wheat or oat bran (optional)

3 tablespoons seeds, such as any combination of flaxseeds or flaxseed

meal, sunflower, pumpkin, sesame, or chia seeds

5 cups mixed nuts and dried fruit, such as any combination of raisins, dates, dried blueberries, unsalted cashews, coconut flakes, or sliced almonds

spices such as cinnamon, cardamom, or nutmeg, to taste (optional)

1. Measure and thoroughly mix all of the ingredients in a large mixing bowl.

2. Transfer the finished mixture to a large, sealed container.

3. Use the dry muesli to make overnight muesli or eat small amounts dry for a snack.

THE POWER OF **Pooping**

Overnight Muesli

Prep time: 5 to 7 minutes plus overnight to refrigerate | Serves: 2 | Fiber Total: 54 to 56 grams

2 cups Dry Muesli (see page 194)

1. Add the muesli to a medium bowl.

2. Pour 1 cup oat milk on the dry muesli mixture and let it sit a for few minutes to soften.

3. Refrigerate overnight.

4. The next morning, top with fresh fruits such as banana, blueberries, or strawberries. Enjoy it for breakfast!

KEY FEATURES OF THIS DISH

- The nutritional value from this meal comes from the many different types of grains in it that have oodles of healthy fiber and complex carbohydrates.

Healthy Burrito with Brown Rice, Beans, and Chicken

Burritos can be both healthy *and* delicious. On top of that, they are easy to prepare! Make yours as simple or as elaborate as you want, but the *key* thing is to make it tasty and healthy. Some people like to buy supersize or standard-size tortillas. This will obviously influence how much you are going to eat, because the larger the tortilla, the more goodies it will hold. Moderation is the key. Enjoy this burrito with a piece of melon or a fresh salad. Incorporate this in your summer menu, or extend it into fall and winter, along with a tasty soup. Buy precooked meat or veggie protein if you want to save time.

**Prep time: 20 minutes | Cook time: 11 minutes |
Serves: 2 | Total Fiber: 30 to 35 grams**

FOR THE SALSA

1 medium tomato, diced (½ cup)

3 tablespoons chopped scallions

1 clove garlic, minced

¼ cup chopped cilantro

2 teaspoons lime juice

salt and pepper, to taste

1 teaspoon finely diced jalapeño pepper

FOR THE BROWN RICE, BEANS, AND CHICKEN

1 cup Seeds of Change organic brown rice and quinoa combo (use cooked brown rice or quinoa as a substitute)

cumin, to taste

garlic powder, to taste

chipotle, to taste

cayenne powder, to taste

salt, to taste

pepper, to taste

2 medium whole-wheat or gluten-free chickpea tortillas

8 ounces cubed chicken or tofu

1 tablespoon olive oil

2 tablespoons scallions

1 cup canned cooked beans of choice, drained

1 tablespoon shredded Mexican 3-cheese blend or jack cheese (optional)

1 tablespoon sour cream or plain yogurt (optional)

2 cups any combination of fresh veggies, such as shredded lettuce or sliced avocado

1. For the salsa: Put the diced tomato, scallions, garlic, and cilantro into a small mixing bowl. Add the lime juice, salt, and jalapeño and mix thoroughly. Set aside.

2. Microwave the rice and quinoa combo according to package instructions, about 90 seconds. If you are using cooked, stand-alone rice or quinoa instead, warm it up so it is ready to use.

3. Sauté the cubed chicken or tofu in the olive oil (while constantly stirring), along with any seasonings you are using (cumin, garlic powder, chipotle or cayenne pepper, salt, and pepper.) For the chicken, sauté over medium-high heat until slightly brown, 5 to 7 minutes. If using tofu, sauté it over medium heat for 3 to 4 minutes. Add the scallions for the last 2 minutes of sautéing for either the chicken or tofu. (Alternatively, you can roast the chicken breast with olive oil, salt, and pepper.)

4. Microwave the tortilla for 60 seconds with a moistened paper towel on top.

5. Add your filling to the tortilla, and be creative! Start with 1 to 2 tablespoons of cooked rice in a narrow line in the center of the tortilla with space on each side, then add the same amount of beans. Now add 2 tablespoons of your protein, veggies, and salsa, and 1 tablespoon of cheese.

6. Now fold each side of the tortilla inward to keep the filling inside, then roll the bottom of the tortilla over the filling while holding your fingers on both the folded sides to secure it as you roll it over to meet the top.

7. Top your burrito with sour cream or yogurt and another tablespoon of salsa if you like to give it a bit more flavor and a little more zing!

8. Repeat steps 3 and 7 for the second burrito.

Optional step: Another option is to nix the tortilla, layer the ingredients in a bowl and—voila—you have your very own "burrito in a bowl." This is a way of cutting carbs if that is important to you. Drizzle some sour cream on top of the salsa.

CHEF BUTTY'S BONUS TIP

To increase your fiber intake, pair your burrito with another fiber-rich food, like a smoothie or a piece of fruit.

KEY FEATURES OF THIS DISH

- In addition to loads of fiber, the chicken (or tofu) contains a lot of protein. This is an ideal dish that exceeds your fiber requirement of 10 grams per meal. Remember, the more fiber you consume, the softer and richer your future poops will be.

- Also loaded with antioxidants, essential vitamins, and complex carbs, this recipe will help keep your gut healthy and happy.

Curried Cubed Chicken Salad

I love spicy, sweet, crunchy, and savory dishes just like my Curried Cubed Chicken Salad. Make it creamy by simply adding a dollop of mayonnaise (organic mayonnaise is fine as long as you don't overdo it).

This tangy salad will perk up your taste buds with such a nice variety of protein, fiber, good fats, and nutrients that your body will thank you by having a dreamy poop!

Serve the curried chicken over a green salad, in a tortilla wrap, with pita bread crackers, or over a bed of quinoa or brown rice. The grapes, nuts, and curry create the perfect balance of flavors.

Prep time: 20 minutes, plus 30 minutes to refrigerate | Cook time: No cook time using precooked chicken | Serves: 2 | Total Fiber: 20 to 26 grams

1 to 2 tablespoons yellow curry powder

½ cup organic mayonnaise

½ apple, diced

½ stalk celery, finely chopped

½ cup halved seedless red or green grapes

1 tablespoon finely chopped green onions

1 tablespoon nuts such as cashew halves, slivered almonds, peanuts, or walnuts

½ cup canned pineapple tidbits, drained

1 tablespoon panko bread crumbs

1 tablespoon cold-pressed, extra-virgin olive oil (optional)

4 ounces cooked chicken breast, cubed (leftover chicken is great)

salt and pepper, to taste

1 cup leafy greens such as spinach, kale, lettuce, arugula

1 slice whole grain or sourdough bread

½ avocado, sliced

1. In a small bowl, mix the yellow curry powder into the mayonnaise and set aside.

2. Place the apple, celery, grapes, green onion, and nuts in a medium bowl. Add salt and pepper to taste.

3. Add the unsweetened pineapple tidbits.

4. Add the panko breadcrumbs to soak up the moisture from the fruits. This is a little trick to help the curry salad hold its shape.

5. Add the curry mayonnaise, olive oil, if using, and cooked chicken to the mixing bowl. Mix thoroughly, making sure the mayonnaise coats all of the ingredients. Season with salt and pepper.

6. Refrigerate for 30 minutes.

7. Place your cold curry salad on a bed of ½ cup of greens or a slice of whole-grain or sourdough bread. Top it off with half of the sliced avocado, and repeat for your remaining serving.

KEY FEATURES OF THIS DISH

- Yellow curry provides good flavor and a little kick, and it has antioxidants and anti-inflammatory properties.

Healthy PB&J Sandwich with Multigrain Bread

This is such a wonderful portable meal. There's hardly any meal prep, just some good-quality whole grain bread, with a generous spread of some smooth or crunchy nut butter, fruit spread, and sliced apples or bananas. It is tasty, healthy, and so easy to make.

Prep time: 15 minutes | Cook time: 0 minutes | Serves: 1 | Total Fiber: 10 to 12 grams

2 slices whole grain wheat bread or whole grain bread of choice

2 to 3 tablespoons raw organic nut butter

1 tablespoon fruit spread or jam of choice

⅓ to ½ cup sliced apple, pear, or banana

1. Toast your bread.

2. Spread your nut butter on each side of the bread, then top it with some jam or fruit spread. I like using fig, strawberry, or raspberry jam since the seeds add a little fiber. There is a scant amount of fiber in jam with seeds in it, under .05 grams per tablespoon.

3. Add the sliced apple, pear, or banana over one slice before topping it with the other piece of bread. Remember to eat any leftover apple or banana so it isn't wasted.

4. Enjoy this with your favorite beverage or at least 8 ounces of water to help wash it down. You can also add another piece of fruit along with your sandwich, or drink some of your high-fiber smoothie for some added fiber.

KEY FEATURES OF THIS DISH

- In total, you have over 10–12 grams of fiber and 8 grams of protein in one healthy sandwich that's a poop favorite!

- Homemade jam or preserves from apricot, berries, or figs contain fewer processed sugars and more from the peels.

Chicken Noodle Vegetable Soup

For another nutritious and satisfying meal, cook an entire chicken and just use parts of it to make this soup. I like to use about 4 chicken thighs and cook them in some organic chicken broth with plenty of veggies to add more flavor.

Cooked vegetables, meat, and herbs give this soup a well-rounded flavor. Make it once a week to ensure you are getting an adequate amount of fiber in your diet. Wait till the soup cools down, then create individual servings in sealable containers.

Prep time: 30 minutes | Cook time: 45 minutes |
Serves: 3 | Total Fiber: 16 to 20 grams

1 yellow onion, chopped

1 to 2 cloves garlic

1 cup chopped celery

1 to 2 tablespoons olive oil

1 teaspoon dried thyme

1 teaspoon ground rosemary

salt and pepper, to taste

12 ounces skinless chicken legs or thighs

4 carrots, cut into bite-sized pieces

2 potatoes, sweet potatoes, parsnips, or turnips, cut into small cubes

1 quart chicken stock

1 cup dry whole grain or vegetable pasta, or 1 can garbanzo or cannellini beans

1. Sauté the onion, garlic, and celery in a 6-quart pot with the olive oil. Add the thyme and rosemary, then add salt and pepper to taste.

2. Brown the chicken in a separate pan, about 5 minutes per side. Drain the fat.

3. Add the chicken, carrots, and potatoes to the onion mixture in the large pot. Pour the chicken stock to cover the contents so they are completely submerged. This allows all the liquid to cook into the ingredients and to soften and flavor everything.

4. Cover with a lid ventilated with a small steam hole and bring to a boil over high heat. Reduce to a simmer and cook for 30 to 45 minutes. During the last 10 minutes of cooking, add the dried pasta and more water as needed to make sure that you have enough liquid to cook it. The noodles will thicken up the soup more. If you are not interested in noodles, use garbanzo or cannellini beans instead.

KEY FEATURES OF THIS DISH

- Soup is easier to digest since cooking helps tenderize the ingredients.

- The broth is helpful in hydrating your body, which helps transport the food in your gut more smoothly.

- After cooking for the allotted time, the meat is so tender it just falls off the bones, and the mixture of vegetables and herbs makes it taste super delicious.

Tomato Mozzarella Basil Salad

In summer, serve this quick, easy dish when fresh basil and tomatoes are readily available. The fresh and flavorful salad provides a zesty zing to your palate and is a wonderful complement to soup, a sandwich, or a slightly heavier meal. It has fiber, protein, good fat, and plenty of vitamins and minerals to keep your body grooving and your poop moving!

**Prep time: 15 minutes, plus 1 hour to chill |
Cook Time: No cooking needed | Serves: 2 |
Total Fiber: 7 to 8 grams**

1½ fresh medium to large heirloom tomatoes, sliced

¼ cup fresh basil leaves, torn or left whole

¼ pound fresh mozzarella cheese, sliced into large chunks

2 teaspoons aged balsamic vinegar

1½ tablespoons cold-pressed extra-virgin olive oil

kosher salt and pepper, to taste

2 slices whole grain wheat bread or 2 slices sourdough bread

1. Arrange the tomatoes, basil leaves, and mozzarella cheese on a platter.

2. Mix the balsamic vinegar and olive oil with some cracked salt and pepper, and drizzle the dressing over the salad.

3. Chill the salad in the refrigerator for 1 hour.

4. Each salad serving should include 1 slice of whole grain wheat or sourdough bread.

KEY FEATURES OF THIS DISH

- Eating whole grains that supply B vitamins, iron, copper, zinc, magnesium, antioxidants, and phyto-chemicals helps the body with disease prevention.

- Tomatoes have lycopene and carotenoids, including beta-carotene, all great antioxidants, along with 1.5 grams of fiber in per tomato.

- Mozzarella cheese is loaded with protein but is also high in fat, so consider using the low-fat variety.

- Olive oil contains omega-3 fatty acids.

DINNER

Oven-Roasted Fish with Polenta and Vegetables

Fish is easy to cook and has many nutritional benefits. Salmon, along with other oily fish like trout, tuna, mackerel, and swordfish, is high in heart-healthy omega-3 fatty acids. Fish doesn't last very long in the fridge, so cook within two days of purchase. While this recipe includes a side dish of polenta, roasted fish is also delicious served with rice, quinoa, or a potato.

Eating fish is easier to digest than denser proteins like meat. Chew slowly and be mindful of any bones. You may even have a glass of wine with it. Food should be about savoring and celebrating the joy of life (and great poops to come).

Prep time: 30 to 45 minutes | Cook time: 19 minutes | Serves: 2 | Total Fiber: 20 to 25 grams

dusting of white flour

salt and pepper

2 (8-ounce) fish fillets of your choice

1 head of broccoli, chopped into florets

1 beet, cut in ½-inch slices

1 carrot, cut in ½-inch slices

1 artichoke heart, cut in ½-inch slices

1 sweet potato, cut in ½-inch slices

1 tomato, cut in ½-inch slices

1 medium zucchini, cut in ½-inch slices

1 medium summer squash, cut in ½-inch slices

1 clove garlic, minced

1 medium mushroom, sliced

1 cup curly-leaf parsley, finely chopped

2 tablespoons cold-pressed extra-virgin olive oil to drizzle over the veggies, plus more to coat the baking sheet

1½ cups premade polenta from a tube, cut into slices

1. Preheat the oven to 400°F.

2. Lightly coat the fish with a dusting of white flour mixed with salt and pepper. This step will help keep your fish moist during the cooking process, and it may even give it some crispy edges.

3. Line a baking sheet with foil, parchment paper, or a heat-resistant silicone mat and spray evenly with olive oil. Place all of the veggies on the lined baking sheet, leaving room for the fish in the middle, as it will be added later for cooking. Spread the herbs over the veggies. Brush, drizzle, or spray olive oil evenly over the seasoned vegetables.

4. Roast the veggies in the oven for 7 to 10 minutes.

5. After the veggies have cooked, place the coated fish with the sliced polenta next to it in the allotted space and bake everything together for 10 minutes. After 10 minutes, pierce the fish with a fork and twist it gently to see if it flakes easily. If so, then it is done, and you can enjoy your delicious creation.

KEY FEATURES OF THIS DISH

- Fish is a healthy protein. Farmed fish is a little higher in omega-3 fatty acids since it is given fortified feed. Some people prefer wild-caught fish, but the farmed fish is more widely available.

- Polenta, a cornmeal that is a complex carbohydrate, is a healthy source of fiber that's not too high in calories and can help you feel fuller longer. One cup of polenta has about 6 grams of fiber. Polenta also has protein and is a gluten-free grain.

- Roasted vegetables give you the fiber to help with constipation. There is no fiber in fish, so pairing it with vegetables is really important. Remember, the darker-color vegetables, such as broccoli, beets, carrots, artichokes, and broccoli rabe, have more fiber.

- There are about 7.4 grams of protein in an average, 4 to 6-ounce serving of tilapia, and a whopping 28 to 42 grams in the same amount of salmon.

Roasted Lemon Herbed Chicken with Brown Rice and Veggies

This is one of my go-to dishes—it's fairly simple to cook and bursts with flavor, plenty of fiber, and lots of protein and nutrients. The lemon slices help tenderize and enhance the flavor of the chicken along with the herbs. A whole roasted chicken can yield plenty of leftovers to make other dishes like Curried Cubed Chicken Salad (page 200); simmer the carcass to provide a base oozing with flavor for Chicken Noodle Vegetable Soup (page 205). Or, use the leftover meat to create an awesome chicken sandwich with greens, tomato, and avocado.

Prep time: 30 to 40 minutes | Cook time: 1 hour | Serves: 4 | Total Fiber: 18 to 21 grams

1 whole medium organic or antibiotic-free roasting chicken

4 carrots, cut into thirds

2 celery stalks, diced

1 whole yellow onion, sliced in large chunks

1 cup broccoli florets

kosher salt and pepper, to taste

2 to 3 tablespoons cold-pressed extra-virgin olive oil, plus more for drizzling

1½ tablespoons herbes de Provence

1 whole lemon, sliced thin

6 cloves garlic

2 cups dry brown rice, cooked

1. Preheat the oven to 400°F. Line a large roasting pan with foil.

2. Put the veggies in a medium-sized bowl, season them with salt and pepper, and drizzle olive oil over them to prevent them from drying out.

3. Mix the olive oil and herbs together in a small bowl.

4. Remove excess fat from chicken. Tuck the lemon slices and the garlic cloves underneath the chicken skin, then pour the herbed oil underneath the skin, saving some to rub over the chicken. This way the entire chicken gets infused with the flavors of the herbs, garlic, and lemon as it cooks.

5. Rub the entire chicken with kosher salt, pepper, and the herbs mixed with olive oil to create a coating over the skin to make it seasoned and crispy. Using a knife, pierce a hole between the joint of the leg and the body so the heat enters the cavity of the chicken.

6. Place the chicken on a roasting rack in a baking pan with the vegetables arranged around it. Put the pan in the oven.

7. Check on the veggies after 30 minutes of cooking time. Flip them to avoid overcooking. Remove them if they are getting overcooked.

8. Cook your brown rice according to the package instructions.

9. After baking for 1 hour, check the internal temperature of the chicken, which should register at or above 160° F. If the temperature is sufficient, remove the chicken and veggies from the oven. Let the chicken cool for 10 minutes, then transfer it to a large cutting board for carving.

10. Skim the fat from the juice using a fat separator. The juice can be poured over the veggies or saved as stock for soup.

11. Place the chicken on a large platter so the juice can ooze onto it. You now have a full meal of protein and fiber to meet your daily requirements, with plenty of leftovers.

KEY FEATURES OF THIS DISH

- Protein from one medium-sized roasted chicken totals a whopping 162 grams. A typical medium-size thigh contains approximately 13 grams of protein, but has no fiber in it.

- When you roast the entire chicken, the juices contain all of the vitamins, minerals, and flavors. There is nothing lost, unlike when you cook only parts of a chicken. The butchers call the residual juice "liquid gold." People say if you are not making chicken stock from the juices, then you are throwing money away! In some special meat markets and delis with rotisserie ovens to roast chickens on site, they sell the chicken stock from the juices for a very high price. So don't be a fool, use the juice and understand you are actually sitting on a pot of gold!

Herb-Roasted Rack of Lamb with Baked Potatoes and Salad

Impress your family and friends with this exquisite meal loaded with rich flavors and packed with protein, fiber, and nutrients. The satisfaction of eating one or two juicy herbed lamb chops is unparalleled, and the portions satisfy you without overeating. The potato has gotten a lot of negative press, but it's the butter, sour cream, bacon bits, and cheese that elevate the fat and calories. If you top the potato minimally, and pair it with the flavorful 4- to 6-ounce portion of meat and salad with a healthy dressing, this meal fulfills the appropriate 40 percent protein and 60 percent fiber needed in a healthy meal. Remember to chew well! This dish fulfills the appropriate 40 percent protein and 60 percent fiber in a meal.

Prep time: 20 to 30 minutes, plus 45 minutes to 2 hours to marinate | Cook time: 30 to 40 minutes, depending on size and desired doneness | Serves: 4 | Total Fiber: 30 to 37 grams

1 (2- to 3-pound) rack of lamb

2 tablespoons fresh or dried rosemary

1 tablespoon dried thyme

3 cloves garlic, minced

1½ teaspoons kosher salt

1½ teaspoons ground pepper

¼ cup cold-pressed extra-virgin olive oil

spinach and/or kale, chopped

¼ cup balsamic vinegar

1 tomato, sliced

4 medium russet potatoes

1 cup cooked beets, diced

1 head romaine, butter, or red leaf lettuce, chopped,

1 medium avocado, sliced into small pieces

½ cup shredded carrots

FOR THE DRESSING:

½ cup olive oil

salt and pepper, to taste

2 tablespoons balsamic vinegar

1. For the lamb: Remove the meat from the fridge and let it rest at room temperature for 20 to 30 minutes; then rinse it with cold water and pat dry. Trim off the surface fat and any silver skin.

2. Prepare your marinade by mixing the rosemary, thyme, fresh garlic, salt, pepper, olive oil, and balsamic vinegar in a 1-gallon ziplock bag.

3. Put the lamb in the bag of marinade, seal tightly, then gently shake the bag to thoroughly coat the meat. Marinate in the fridge for 45 minutes to 2 hours.

4. Preheat the oven to 350°F.

5. Using a fork, pierce the potatoes with several holes, then place them on the oven rack. No need to wrap in foil. Put the potatoes in the oven and set a timer for 25 minutes.

6. With gloves on, carefully remove the marinated lamb from the bag and put it in the roasting pan. Bake for 30 to 40 minutes.

7. When your potatoes have been baking for about 25 minutes, check for doneness by piercing one in the middle with a sharp knife. If there is no resistance, they are done and can be removed. If not, then let them bake a few more minutes before checking again.

8. Check the internal temperature of the lamb with a meat thermometer after it has cooked for 20 to 25 minutes. Insert the thermometer in the thickest part of the meat at least ½ inch deep. The temperature should be 125°F if you like it rare, 130°F for medium rare, and 145°F for well done.

9. After the meat has reached the desired internal temperature, turn off the oven, partially open the door, and let the meat rest in the warm oven for 5 to 10 minutes as it will continue to cook internally. After it has rested, remove it from the oven to cool a few more minutes before carving. Be careful not to overcook the meat or it will dry out and may get tougher.

10. To make the salad, place the greens, beets, tomato, avocado, and carrots together in a bowl and toss, then refrigerate until the main course is ready. Then mix the salad dressing in a small bowl and dress the salad.

11. Once the lamb has rested and cooled, slice it into chops; divide the chops and potatoes between four dinner plates, portion the salad into four bowls, and enjoy your elegant meal.

KEY FEATURES OF THIS DISH

- Lamb is high in protein, iron, vitamin B-12, and zinc. Even though you can see the fat on the surface, the meat is less marbled with it, and so relatively lean. More often than beef, lamb is grass-fed, which is nutritionally superior to grain-fed and avoids a long list of unpleasant additives.

- Although russet potatoes often get a bad rap due to the carbs, they are loaded with fiber, vitamins, and minerals. Most of the fiber in potatoes comes from the skin, which also contains many minerals and fiber. Potatoes also contain vitamin C and gut-friendly starch that can be helpful in keeping your stools bound together.

BUTTY'S BONUS TIP

A nice salad accompanying the main course can add as much as 20 grams of fiber to your meal!

Savory Meatless Cornmeal-Crust Pizza with Baked Figs

Premade cornmeal pizza crust doesn't make you feel nearly as bloated as flour pizza. But if you are on a gluten-free diet, check the labels, as some versions contain wheat flour. I personally like the Vicolo brand crust.

If you want to make a healthy pizza with fresh dark purple California mission figs that is full of antioxidants and fiber, blended with the sweetness of sautéed onions, this meatless pizza is for you.

Prep time: 15 minutes | Cook time: 12 to 15 minutes | Serves: 2 | Total Fiber: 18 to 20 grams

1 sweet yellow Maui onion, sliced

1 cup chopped fresh kale leaves

1 tablespoon cold-pressed extra-virgin olive oil

salt and pepper, to taste

1 teaspoon herbes de Provence, divided

10 fresh, ripe Black Mission figs, sliced in halves or thirds

1 (8.5-inch) premade cornmeal pizza crust

½ cup shredded white cheddar cheese

½ cup feta cheese (optional)

3 tablespoons goat cheese, preferably in a log form from Laura Chenel, mashed

2 tablespoons whole milk

1. Preheat the oven to 425°F.

2. In a large pan, sauté the onion and kale in the olive oil with salt, pepper, and half of the herbes de Provence for 10 minutes. Place the sautéed onions on top of the premade cornmeal pizza crust.

3. Add the kale on top of the sautéed onions, then add the figs, seed side up to caramelize, giving them a sweet crusty texture.

4. Sprinkle the shredded white cheddar cheese and feta, if using, on top of the bed of figs.

5. Place the pizza on an aluminum or silicone baking sheet and bake at 435°F for 12 to 15 minutes, until the cheese and toppings look slightly brown.

6. For the final touch, in a microwave-safe bowl, briefly mix the goat cheese with the milk then heat in the microwave on low for about 30 seconds. Stir the cheese and milk into a creamy consistency.

7. Drizzle the creamy melted cheese over the pizza and enjoy!

KEY FEATURES OF THIS DISH

- Unexpected fruit like figs mixed with onions and cheese actually taste great on a pizza! Figs are loaded with fiber. Figs have a high natural sugar content similar to prunes. The natural sugar helps soften your poops and the seeds act like insoluble fiber.

- The protein from this dish comes from the cheese, along with 4 more grams from the pizza crust. The whole finished pizza has 10 to 17 grams of protein, along with as much as 20 grams of fiber, depending on the amount of ingredients you use. A salad with the meal adds more fiber.

- Drink water or a healthy beverage with your meal to add more moisture to your gut and increase motility. The resulting soft stool will be more easily processed by the colon to move it along the poop chute.

Shrimp with Grains and Veggies

This entire dinner dish sits in a bowl filled with layers of yummy ingredients and special toppings. You can use whole grain rice or a grain of your choice, such as quinoa or barley, available in microwavable pouches or bowls that are heated in 90 seconds and ready to eat.

This easy dish is delicious and elegant, and will satisfy your hunger without making you feel stuffed. The greatest benefit of this dish is—you guessed it—it's very poop-friendly!

Prep time: 5 to 20 minutes | Cook time: 5 to 10 minutes | Serves: 1 | Total Fiber: 18 to 21 grams

1 green onion, chopped

½ cup chopped bell pepper

2 tablespoons cold-pressed extra-virgin olive oil

1 pat of butter

salt and pepper, to taste

6 to 8 medium shrimp, with or without tails

1 tablespoon grated ginger, chopped

1 to 2 cloves garlic. chopped

1 tablespoon gluten-free tamari sauce

1 teaspoon sesame oil

zest and juice of 1 navel orange

¼ cup warm water

1 tablespoon cornstarch

1 cup microwaveable brown rice or cooked quinoa

1 cup frozen edamame, defrosted, for garnish

½ cup avocado, for garnish

¼ cup alfalfa sprouts, for garnish

1 tablespoon sesame seeds

1. In a 10-inch nonstick skillet, sauté the onion and bell pepper in the olive oil and butter. Add salt and pepper. Cook over medium heat for 2 to 3 minutes.

2. Add the shrimp, ginger, and garlic to the pan and sauté, turning the shrimp with tongs after a minute or two. Shrimp cook quickly, in about 5 minutes, and should be a light pink color when done. You can buy frozen or fresh shrimp shelled so you have less work when you eat them. Some people like the shells left on when cooking since it gives the shrimp more taste and keeps the meat moist.

3. Mix the gluten-free tamari with the sesame oil in a large cup and set aside.

4. Pour the orange juice with zest in the pan with shrimp and other ingredients, then add the cornstarch, ¼ cup of warm water, honey, and the tamari mix while stirring vigorously to a thick consistency, about 2 minutes.

5. Heat the grains in a bowl, then place the shrimp mixture on top.

6. Garnish with the edamame, alfalfa sprouts, sliced avocado, and sesame seeds. Now, you're ready to enjoy this delightful dish!

KEY FEATURES OF THIS DISH

- The shrimp is packed with omega-3s, about 15 grams of high-quality protein, and other nutrients.

WEEK-AT-A-GLANCE MEAL SCHEDULE AND TABLE

The following one-week, at-a-glance meal schedule that includes total fiber amounts should give you a template for planning your meals. You can also make your own meal schedule, filling it in with fiber-rich foods of your choice.

BREAKFAST

- Fruit Smoothies (page 182)
- Nurse Wong's Morning Staple: Oatmeal (page 185)
- Overnight Chia Seed Pudding (page 187)
- Overnight Oats (page 190)
- Muesli and Overnight Muesli (page 192)

LUNCH

- Healthy Burrito with Brown Rice, Beans, and Chicken (page 196)
- Curried Cubed Chicken Salad (page 200)
- Healthy PB&J Sandwich with Multigrain Bread (page 203)
- Chicken Noodle Vegetable Soup (page 205)
- Tomato Mozzarella Basil Salad (page 208)

DINNER

- Oven-Roasted Fish with Polenta and Vegetables (page 210)

- Roasted Lemon Herbed Chicken with Brown Rice and Veggies (page 213)

- Herb-Roasted Rack of Lamb with Baked Potatoes and Salad (page 217)

- Savory Meatless Cornmeal-Crust Pizza with Baked Figs (page 222)

- Shrimp with Grains and Veggies (page 225)

The fiber figures on the following chart will vary depending on personal preference and added ingredients.

	Breakfast	Snack	Lunch	Snack	Dinner	Total fiber
Monday	Fruit Smoothie (6 g) Morning Staple Oatmeal (7.5 g)	Apple (3.5 g)	Healthy Burrito w/ Brown Rice, Beans, and Chicken (17.5 g)	Herbal tea w/ oat milk (1 g)	Oven-Roasted Fish w/ Polenta and Vegetables (12.5 g)	48 g
Tuesday	Fruit Smoothie (6 g) Overnight Oats (13.5 g)	Remainder of smoothie	Curried Cubed Chicken Salad w/ 1 slice whole wheat bread (13 g)	Tangerine (1.3 g)	Roasted Lemon Herbed Chicken w/ Brown Rice and Veggies (5 g)	38.8 g

Wednesday	Fruit Smoothie (6 g) Overnight Chia Seed Pudding (8.5 g)	Herbal tea or caffeinated tea w/oat milk (1 g)	Healthy PB&J Sandwich w/ Multigrain Bread (11 g) and the remainder of the smoothie	Banana (3.1 g)	Herb-Roasted Rack of Lamb w/ Baked Potatoes, and Salad (14.5 g)	44.1 g
Thursday	Fruit Smoothie (6 g) Overnight Oats (13.5 g)	Remainder of smoothie	Chicken Noodle Vegetable Soup (8 g)	Oatmeal cookie (1 g)	Savory Meatless Cornmeal-Crust Pizza w/ Baked Figs (9.3 g) 1½ cups green salad (1.2 g)	39 g
Friday	Overnight Muesli w/ oat milk (28 g) Banana (3.1 g)	Fruit Smoothie (6 g)	Tomato Mozzarella Basil Salad (4 g)	Apple (3.5 g) and oatmeal cookie (1 g)	Shrimp w/ Grains and Veggies (21 g)	66.6 g
Saturday	Fruit Smoothie (6 g) Overnight Chia Seed Pudding (8.5 g)	Herbal tea or coffee w/oat milk (1 g)	Healthy Burrito w/ Brown Rice, Beans, and Chicken w/ salsa (17.5 g)	Tangerine (1.3 g)	Oven-Roasted Fish w/ Polenta and Vegetables (12.5 g)	46.8 g

THE POWER OF *Pooping*

Sunday	Fruit Smoothie (6 g) Morning Staple Oatmeal/ fruit/Nuts (7.5 g)	Remainder of smoothie + 1 hard-boiled egg	Curried Cubed Chicken Salad w/ 1 slice whole-grain toast (13 g)	1 cup of popcorn (1 g)	Savory Meatless Cornmeal-Crust Pizza w/Baked Figs (9.3 g) 1½ cups green salad (4.5 g)	41.3 g

As you can see, there are many components to eating healthy, including your budget and time for meal planning and preparation. Use the above template as a starting point on your journey to better gut health. It is by no means set in stone, particularly if you have special dietary needs due to a medical condition, or if you are vegetarian or vegan (if you are, your poops should be fine with all the fiber you eat).

Whether you have an exacerbating medical condition that limits your dietary choices, you like to eat more foods that align with your culture, or you like more variety in your meals, feel free to be creative with the recipes in this book to better meet your health needs, cultural needs, and personal tastes. And don't forget that the most important aspect of making dietary and lifestyle changes is the motivation and self-discipline to improve your gut and overall health in order to fully understand and appreciate the power of pooping!

Although pooping is a topic that some people consider private or even offensive, thousands of us suffer from gut or poop-related problems every day. It is my hope that you've discovered some helpful information as well as a little humor during your reading of *The Power of Pooping.* If any part of this book has given you some insight into your own poop issues or helped you begin to make changes to improve your gut health, thank you for being honest enough with yourself to recognize the need for action. Feel free to share your interest and enthusiasm for *The Power of Pooping* with anyone you know who might benefit from the insights and information contained within these pages.

Have a great poop day!

Nurse Wong

RESOURCES

WEBSITES

Harvard Health Publishing

https://www.health.harvard.edu

A Harvard University online health magazine for people who want to know about everything related to health. A very informative newsletter is available with a subscription.

Mayo Clinic, "Constipation"

https://www.mayoclinic.org/diseases-conditions/constipation/symptoms-causes/syc-20354253

An excellent resource that explores the causes and treatment for constipation in clear, accessible terms.

National Institute of Diabetes and Digestive and Kidney Diseases, "Constipation"

https://www.niddk.nih.gov/health-information/digestive-diseases/constipation

A great resource for using a constipation protocol, along with information on other digestive issues.

Nutrition.gov, "Fats"

https://www.nutrition.gov/topics/whats-food/fats

Another US government website to help you learn what dietary fats do for the body, how much fat is recommended per day, and the fat content in in popular foods.

USDA MyPlate, "Print Materials"

https://www.myplate.gov/resources/print-materials

A US government site for the public to read up on a multitude of topics related to good nutrition, including how we are teaching nutrition to school children, how children eat, and nutritional milestones.

US Food and Drug Administration (FDA), "Consumers"

https://www.fda.gov/food/resources-you-food/consumers

This website provides valuable information on the nutritional content of all types of foods, including how to understand and use nutrition facts labels.

BOOKS

Freuman, Tamara Duker. *The Bloated Belly Whisperer: A Nutritionist's Ultimate Guide to Beating Bloat and Improving Digestive Wellness*. St. Martin's Press, 2018.

The author is a nutritionist who provides excellent information on which foods can help with bloat issues. Many of my patients have read the book and found it very informative.

Wexner, Steven D., and Graeme S. Duthie, editors. *Constipation: Etiology, Evaluation, and Management*, 2nd ed. Springer, 2006.

This very useful book is a reference source for the medical profession.

López-Alt, J. Kenji. *The Food Lab: Better Home Cooking through Science*. W. W. Norton & Company, 2015.

This is a very informative book about cooking and the science of how to treat food to get the best nutrition out of it.

ABOUT THE AUTHORS

Susan Wong, RN, BSN, aka Nurse Wong, is a graduate of the University of California–San Francisco (UCSF) School of Nursing. In her forty-plus years as a nurse, she has served patients at UCSF in a variety o

f settings, including surgical, dialysis, and colorectal. In 1999 she was asked to help with the development of a ground-breaking UCSF colorectal clinic.

Because of her ability to effectively listen and empathize with the beloved patients she treats, Nurse Wong has been affectionately dubbed the "The Rear Admiral" and the "Butt Whisperer" by her coworkers. She has participated in work-shops all across the US, as well as in the Netherlands and Great Britain. She has won several service awards of excellence for contributions to her patient population and is rated one of the top providers at her medical center. In May of 2020, she was interviewed for an article on the use of bidets in the *Smithsonian Magazine*. Also in May of 2020, she launched *Butt Talks TV* on YouTube with the goal of reaching people around the globe with bowel-related issues and demystifying the taboo surrounding poop health. Though still in its infancy, *Butt Talks TV* already has a fast-growing subscribership along with further plans for expansion.

On a personal note, Nurse Wong was one of only five Chinese Americans out of the 140 in her nursing class which, at the time, was a cultural breakthrough. After the passing of her husband in 2003, she raised her son Julien, now a budding entrepreneur. Her first language is Cantonese, and she is also fluent in French. She loves to cook for family and friends using the many herbs grown year-round in her lovely San Francisco patio garden.

John Rietcheck, MA, AuD, is a clinical audiologist with a master's degree from the University of Kansas and a doctorate from Salus University's College of Audiology. He recently retired from the San Francisco VA Health Care System after twenty-nine years in hearing health care. He's worked as a reporter for the *Red Rock News* in Sedona, Arizona, and served as an editor of newsletters for local nonprofit organizations for a combined twenty years in both Topeka, Kansas, and San Francisco, California.

John met Susan Wong through a mutual connection, and they soon became fast friends. Although they worked in different domains, their work with patients in the health-care arena provided them a common bond. When Susan and

Julien asked John if he would like to write scripts for *Butt Talks TV* and later contribute his skills to this book, it seemed like a natural transition from all his years of writing in both official and unofficial capacities.

In his personal life, John is a singer and songwriter who has written and recorded many of his songs on two music albums. Now a resident of northern Nevada near Lake Tahoe, he enjoys cooking, reading, hiking, and playing disc golf.